And the GREATEST *of These*

A Novel by Joe Pritchard

COVENANT
COMMUNICATIONS
NASHVILLE, TN

BIRDCAGE
www.midnightbirdcage.com

BIRDCAGE
www.midnightbirdcage.com

For Mom and Pop...

And now these three remain: faith, hope and love. But the greatest of these is love.

I Corinthians 13:13 (NIV).

A T FIRST GLANCE THEY SEEMED like all the rest. All the rest, that is, in a psychiatric emergency room.

I make my meager living in one of Nashville's busiest mental health thoroughfares. The white collars who sign my bi-monthly checks call me an assessment specialist, a fancy name for a crisis counselor. They give me a badge with my mug shot, tell me to admit all paying customers, and pray that I stay in touch with reality along the way. Sometimes I wonder which side of the assessment desk I belong on.

On any given day, I have the twelve-hour pleasure of discussing the game of life with the homeless and the hopeless both young and old, rich and poor, including physically and sexually traumatized kids, women, men, and, sad to say, the newest members of the abuse club — the elderly. From street-hustling hookers selling their souls for one more hit off that crack pipe to uptown alcoholics craving another shot to sustain their lives; from Alzheimer's patients lost in some fog of a life to overdose victims way down on life to schizophrenics who see things in a different light, the psychiatric soul train never ceases to choke and chug its way along the bruised and battered halls of Faith General, Nashville's oldest hospital.

And heaven forbid we exclude our bipolar friends. There's nothing like manic Mondays at Faith General and the frenzied tirades of spastic females demanding admission to our stress disorders unit. I'm partial to our end-of-the-month Mad Dog Mondays when the Music City's finest depressed drunks, having consumed all of their disability dough, check-in at our second floor bed and breakfast, also known as our inpatient dual treatment program. The Faith General Hilton, as it's known on the streets, continental breakfast included. We call them frequent flyers. Truth be known, these ol' walls would collapse if not for them, and our legion of foreign psychiatrists would not be driving those fine Mercedes if it weren't for the recidivist revolving door.

It's not just the addicts who come and go. Our revolving door also includes a steady flow of truly mentally ill folk who, after taking their prescribed medicines for two months, stop taking the magic potions that keep the demons at bay, only to see Jesus in their Cornflakes again or hear voices telling them to jump off the Cumberland River Bridge.

I don't mean to sound calloused. It's just that day after depressing day I hear their stories when, in reality, I only need about five minutes to determine whether or not they warrant admission to one of our six psychiatric units. Most, however, want to ramble on, and they do until I gingerly cut them off. Speed is critical in my job as an assessment specialist. If I spend too much time with one case, the ER backs up and everyone becomes testy, especially the docs and nurses who don't like dealing with our patients. I don't blame them. I don't like dealing with psychiatric patients who have medical problems.

I still have a heart for those who genuinely want and need help. I just know how to keep my emotions at bay and do my job with the precision and aloofness of a brain surgeon. I do care, but I don't. It's an art form: rapid-fire manipulation of multiple systems to quickly get them treatment while making each one feel cared for. I tell the rookie staff it's the closest we'll ever get to Hollywood.

And so it was with John and Maggie Dalton. They weren't the first elderly couple I had assessed and subsequently admitted (one or the other) to our geriatric psychiatric unit. I'm uncomfortable dealing with that population. Too much medical and way too close to home and a myriad of memories about Mom and Pop. Escorting couples down that unpredictable geri-psych hallway was a task I often found a way to avoid.

It was past my clock-out time, when I should have been home sipping bourbon and self-stimulating the night away with my TV buttons, that I saw Maggie Dalton stroke John's haggard face. That picture ripped right through my Hollywood persona to the core of my soul. In that instant, I saw Mom stroking Pop's deceased face and fighting back tears, the agonized, little-girl-lost look in her hazel eyes a replica of Maggie's eyes that night.

It was a line I'd vowed never to cross again – unconditional love of another human being.

chapter one

THE POLICE BROUGHT HIM IN handcuffed, the royal treatment usually reserved for those truly deranged or violent. Within minutes, ER was calling psych assessments.

"Are you expecting a patient?"

"Nope," I snapped, glancing at the referral board. "What have you got?" I was hoping for a drunk or a psychotic female, just someone I could quickly assess and pass on. The sun was setting, ER was packed, and a pint of Jack Daniel's was calling my name.

"Seventy-six year old delusional male," replied the ER triage nurse. "I told the cop to take him on to the back and put him in one of the seclusion rooms until you got there."

"I don't need this..."

"His wife's with him and pretty upset. Can you talk to her?"

I slammed the phone down and grabbed an assessment form. Before I could get out of our broom-closet office, the phone rang again. The drunk I longed for was on the line, plastered, yearning to tell me his life story. I cut him off. "We don't send vans out to pick people up. You make it to the liquor store every day. Surely you can find someone..."

"You sorry son of a bitch," he stammered and hung up.

"Get a life," I mumbled as I scurried out the door and down the drab Faith General ER hallway. I placed my security key into the wall lock that activated the steel-enforced security doors leading into the back portion of the ER known as the psychiatric assessments department. Dead ahead, approximately thirty feet, a sheriff's deputy stood blocking the doorway to one of two seclusion rooms, both twelve-by-twelve, identical, beige boxes with built-in mattresses and mounted cameras, allowing staff to monitor patients sleeping, pacing, urinating, stripping, or if truly agitated and combative, locked in for safety's sake. On either side of the seclusion rooms were two barren interview rooms, each with a smattering of mix-and-match hand-me-down chairs with club-like arms dying to break free and into the hands of some deranged or drunken patient threatening to bash my skull if I don't let him out to smoke.

The deputy saw me and stepped into the hallway.

"What's up with this one?" I asked as I visually assessed the patient, who sat stoically in handcuffs. His wavy white hair was neatly combed, his blue Polo shirt appropriately buttoned, his Dockers creased, shoes clean, socks matched and actually pulled up, revealing no skin. Definitely not disheveled or unkempt as was often the case with demented and delusional geriatric patients.

The deputy glanced back at the elderly man. "He took a swing at me, not to mention what he tried to do to his wife."

"She call you guys out?"

"A neighbor called 911. Said she saw him on their back deck threatening his wife with a butcher knife. She doesn't know what's going on. It's like he turned into a madman of sorts for no apparent reason."

I nodded to the deputy and stepped into the seclusion room. "Mr. Dalton..." I looked into his eyes, hoping to make some type of connection. "Mr. Dalton, my name is Michael. I'm going to ask you a few questions, okay? See if we can get you some help."

He looked up and straight through me as if I didn't exist.

"Mr. Dalton, do you know where you are?" I asked, easing my weight back on my left leg.

He looked my way, only this time something clicked. "You're the one!" he cried, lunging full force.

I pivoted back, providing the deputy plenty of time and room to bear-hug the wild-eyed man back down onto the mat.

"What's next?" the cop asked with a told-you-so smile.

"Guess I'll try the wife," I said. "Security is on the way. Thanks for helping us out."

I keyed the wall lock, hustled back down the ER hallway and entered our meet-and-greet triage room. I took a deep breath and opened the door leading out to the ER waiting room. "Mrs. Dalton?" I called out to the dead-eyed mass of faces that always turned my way, yearning for their names to be called. I scanned the room, looking no one in the eye, all the while hoping that the wife of my patient would appear and fast.

"Yes!" A voice cried out among the mumbling throng.

I saw a frail hand rise among the standing room only crowd near the main entrance. "I'm Ms. Dalton," she announced and walked across that dingy waiting room floor with an air of down-home sophistication and humility, an endangered combination these days. "Maggie Dalton," she said to me, extending a firm handshake and a deep gaze into my eyes that froze me for a split-second. "Do you need to speak to me about John?"

"Yes ma'am," I said, yearning for a brief interview and a Medicare card, knowing her husband needed to be hospitalized on our geriatric psychiatric unit for observation, if nothing else. If he had regular Medicare, I wouldn't have to call and fight to obtain the authorization to admit, as was always the case with HMO Medicare, Medicaid and private insurances. I could simply admit him once I completed all of the paperwork, paged the on-call psychiatrist, and gave verbal report to the unit RN. I still had a shot at clocking out in forty minutes.

With the ER packed and our interview rooms occupied, I led her to the grief room, a postage stamp space with an oversized cloth couch, vinyl loveseat, and plastic table barely big enough to hold a hideous lamp and phone. The grief room was ER's designated area for families and loved ones of patients who'd died for whatever reason. It didn't happen that often. Faith General's ER spilled over most days with far more wayward souls than heart attack victims.

I directed Maggie to the couch and watched her sink into its gaudy green-plaid upholstery. She took a deep breath and sank even further, the wind slowing fading from her sails.

"Are you okay?" I asked. I was nervous. I was always nervous around elderly patients and especially their spouses. What do you say to them? *Gee, I'm sorry your husband is delusional and urinating in the sink. I can empathize with what you must be feeling.* How can I even begin to understand what it's like to live with an elderly, delusional spouse? I couldn't live with a 37-year-old sane one.

Maggie Dalton looked up and smiled, as graceful a look as I've ever seen. "What was your name?" she asked.

"Michael."

"Yes, Michael, I'm hanging in there." She looked down, as if fighting back tears.

My gut told me she wasn't about to cry. The look in her hazel eyes — an intense yet mellow look — revealed too much intestinal fortitude and class to lose it with a total stranger.

"What happened today?" I asked, still counting on a quick interview.

She sighed. "Fifty-six years..." She closed her eyes for a brief moment. Her silver gray hair was cropped close to her head, giving her a look much younger than her seventy-something years on this earth.

"May I call you Maggie?" I asked, readjusting my Wal-Mart reading glasses.

"Fifty-six years..." She looked at me with an eerie smile.

"Maggie?" I tried to re-focus her attention. "I need to ask you..."

"Yes," she interrupted.

"Yes?"

"Please call me Maggie."

"Maggie, what happened at your home today that the police had to come out?"

"Michael, are you married?" she asked, ignoring my question altogether.

"Divorced," I reluctantly replied.

"Any kids?"

"One boy. Actually, he's a young man now," I said. "Twenty-one years old."

"Are you close to him?"

That one caught me off guard, as if I was the psych patient and she was assessing me. I stared down at the blank assessment attached to my old clipboard, not wanting to face her motherly wrath.

She waited on me to look up. "Well, are you?" she demanded.

"No, I'm not." I reshuffled my clipboard, hoping again to redirect her and regain my rattled composure.

"Don't let this happen to you before you get things right with your son," she said, her eyes fierce. "Do you understand Michael? Get things right with your son before it's too late."

"Yes ma'am," I replied, "I will." Suddenly, I was the deflated one. Maggie's words stung me, much like my Mom's declaration the day I left Knoxville, challenging me to get off my pity pot and make things right with "my boy," or I'd live to regret it.

"Before I tell you what happened today," she said, again waiting on me to make eye contact, "please allow me a few minutes to tell you a story. Or, if that's asking too much…"

"No…" I laid my clipboard on the table, trumped for the time being. "Not at all."

My best friend, Jack Daniels, would have to wait.

chapter two

"I'LL NEVER FORGET THE FIRST time I saw him," Maggie said, sitting erect, a smile on her face. "My goodness, he was a handsome man in that uniform. He waltzed into my father's store and my heart stopped."

I nodded and smiled, glancing at my watch, dying to clock out and head home where I could drink in solitude. And yet, for some reason, I couldn't bring myself to cut her off. I'd done it before. Stopped or redirected their geriatric babbling. In a nice way, of course. But, not this time. Not with Maggie Dalton. Those poignant eyes and her motherly demand to get my parenting house in order had jolted me, as if Mom were speaking to me through this woman.

"There I was the eighteen-year-old daughter of hardworking Southern Baptist parents. I was smitten!" She chuckled, a big grin on her face. "Oh, how they despised him at first. We were married on April 27, 1956, in the same church where I was baptized as a little girl. " She sighed and fell back into the couch.

I started to stand. She shot me a look that made it all too clear she wasn't finished yet. I eased back in my seat.

She scooted up to the edge of the old couch. "Fifty-six years…"

I leaned forward, intrigued with fifty-six years of anything, much less what appeared to be a happy loving marriage.

"We celebrated our fifty-sixth wedding anniversary last month." Maggie gently twirled the silver wedding band on her finger. "John surprised me."

"What did he do?" I settled back and crossed my leg.

"He took me back to the little church where we'd said our vows. I asked him why all the hoopla and he looked at me like I was crazy."

"What did he say?" I stroked my chin and nodded.

She smiled, eager to continue. "He reminded me that he'd promised to keep his word. I was still in the dark until he mentioned Joe DiMaggio and his 56-game hitting streak."

"The Yankee Clipper," I said with a smile.

"You know him too?"

I felt a lump in my throat.

"Michael?" Maggie held her gaze.

"He was one of my Dad's heroes," I replied, unable to sustain eye contact. "Mom too. She was... is a huge baseball fan."

She glanced at her ring, then back at me as she clutched her hand. "John always told me that if DiMaggio could do the seemingly impossible for fifty-six straight games, then the least he could do was give me fifty-six faithful years of marriage. How ironic, huh?"

I nodded, memories of my parents in the stands for *every* home baseball game I *ever* played, including my last at the University of Tennessee, a season-long hitting slump that dashed my lifetime dream of playing a kids' game for a living.

"One month later," she broke into my thoughts, "and here we sit in this emergency room. Oh, I could see the changes in him — the memory loss and forgetfulness, the bad dreams during daytime naps — but he was keeping it together pretty well. And physically, he was doing fine. Heck, we're doing fine."

She sat upright. "For two old birds in our seventies, we're doing quite well. I wonder…"

"What?" I asked.

"He's such a man of honor." She stroked her ring again, appearing deep in thought.

I remained silent.

She turned her attention back to me. "He always told me it was the way DiMaggio carried himself, a man of class and integrity. Through thick and thin, he was the same. Always there, always dependable, and willing to give it his best." Her eyes intensified, her voice strong and firm. "That's what John meant when he said he would match DiMaggio's streak."

I nodded, wondering where I'd gone so painfully wrong with my marriage and life. Wondering where I'd gone wrong with getting out of this room and home.

"The Good Lord blest me when John Robert Dalton walked through that country store fifty-six years ago," Maggie proclaimed. "There'll be no sending him to the bullpen as long as I'm alive." She glanced skyward and pointed. "You hear me up there Mr. DiMaggio?" She braced her right hand on the old couch, and stood, as dignified and elegant as any woman I'd ever seen.

I stood with her in that tiny grief room, our eyes meeting.

"Thank-you Michael, for listening."

I acknowledged her and smiled, taken back by the emotions stirring inside me. "Sounds like the two of you have had a wonderful life together."

"We've been blest," she said. "Has it always been easy? No, in some ways, anything but."

"You didn't mention kids," I said as I eased the door open. "Do you have children?"

She stopped in the doorway and turned to face me. "That's

18

why you have to help me, Michael. Help me with John before it's too late."

"Too late for what?" I asked.

"It's his only son." She clasped my forearm, reeling me in. "Our son."

"What is it?" I asked, gently pulling back.

"Can I see John now? Please, just let me talk to him."

"Maggie, he's not well. He's..."

"Please..."

chapter three

WE EDGED OUR WAY DOWN the hectic ER hallway towards the psych ER area. I saw our security guard loitering at the nursing station, leaving me to wonder who was watching John in the seclusion room. I had Maggie wait in the hallway while I hustled over to him.

"Pete, you watching the guy in seclusion?"

"He's been sitting on the mat, calm as could be," he said. "Staff knows to call me."

"Sounds good." I keyed the wall lock and held the steel-enforced door open, expecting, as I felt Maggie's watchful eyes, to see John in the seclusion room. "He ain't sittin' now," I muttered, recalling last month's eighty-one-year-old delusional farmer who'd slipped out behind unsuspecting kitchen staff and made it to the parking lot before anyone realized what had happened. Not wanting to alarm Maggie, I smiled reassuringly and slid back over to the cramped ER nursing station.

"Any ideas where the guy in seclusion is?" I asked.

"He's your patient," snapped Susan, the second shift RN. "You tell me."

"No," I fired back, trying to hide my frustration. "We've had this discussion. Until medically cleared, they're your patients and your responsibility too."

"Look, Michael..." She gestured at eight treatment rooms overflowing with patients and their families, the early evening run of sniffles and moans filling the cramped, rush-hour-like ER hallway.

"Michael?"

I recognized the voice. It was Maggie.

As I turned to face her, the ER hallway bathroom door opened.

"Hey Honey!" John called out, beaming with joy as he lunged towards her, Maggie never hesitating as she fell into his arms. She looked up at him and stroked his smiling face, their eyes locked on one another, oblivious to the chaos whizzing by them. I stood beside them, redirecting traffic, lost somewhere between adolescent flashbacks of my parents embracing and knowing that I had to get some answers.

I led them back behind locked doors and safely past a manic female ranting and pacing. I eased the interview room door closed and got down to business.

"John," I turned towards him, "do you recall meeting me earlier?"

He studied my face. "No, can't say that I do."

"I'm Michael, from the assessment office."

"Assessments?" He cocked his head to one side.

"It's okay, dear." Maggie touched his hand. "Michael's here to help."

I leaned forward. "John, do you know where you are?"

"At Faith General, getting a check-up."

"A check-up?" I asked, playing dumb, turning towards Maggie, my eyes requesting that she let him answer.

He turned towards her. "She was worried about me. Said I wasn't acting myself, and I should see a doctor. Are you the doctor?"

"No, I work with the ER doctor, assisting him in finding out how we can help you."

"Help me for what?" he snapped, agitated again, the veins in his neck bulging.

I glanced at Maggie, this time my eyes asking for help. She obliged.

"Honey..." She caressed his hand. "Do you remember what happened just a little while ago at home?" Her hand trembled as she reached up and gently turned his face towards her. "Do you remember when you woke up from your afternoon nap?"

"Not really," he said, succumbing to her gentle touch. "I had a bad dream, I think."

"What happened in your dream?" I asked.

"I'm not sure exactly," he said. "Seems like I was chasing someone through the house. A robber, I think." John turned back to Maggie, patting her hand. "He was after you."

She glanced at me, her eyes begging me to back off.

I obliged, an eerie sense of allegiance to Maggie, and to John, building. They reminded me so much of my parents, especially after Pop had retired and he and Mom had the time to take day trips and leisurely hang out together. He dropped dead at home from a heart attack a year later, leaving me to wish I'd spent more time with him. Mom too. Pop had mellowed out and was more approachable then, and what did I do?

John shifted in his chair.

"You feel okay now?" I asked.

"A little tired, but I'm all right. When do I see the doctor?"

"Soon. I've just got a few more questions to ask," I said, nodding at Maggie.

He responded surprisingly well, with no current evidence of delusions or hallucinations, yet, I knew a life-threatening incident had occurred only a few hours earlier.

"John," I patted him on his shoulder, "hang in there for a few more minutes, okay? Let me see what I can do to get the ER doc over here." I nodded to Maggie. "You got a second?"

She was reluctant to leave his side but consented, reassuring him that everything was okay and she'd return shortly. I let Security Pete know to monitor John and directed Maggie out the ambulance entrance.

"Used to be my favorite time of day," she said, gazing westward at the surrounding hills, twinkling street lights and twilight sky as it slowly shed its pink and purple hue.

"Always been my favorite," I said as I led her to a small grassy plot with a picnic table directly across from the ambulance bay. "Nothing like that last tinge of daylight, a thin layer of clouds, stars to the east." I sat down across from her. "The greatest light show on earth."

Maggie turned back towards the western sky, her silhouette reminding me of Mom long after Pop had passed. "John and I used to walk at dusk…" She looked away.

"What is it?"

"John's fading from me. He's…" She abruptly stood, glancing towards the ER. "We should go check on him."

I stood next to her. "I want the best for the two of you, I truly do. But I'm concerned. I know you didn't allow the police to bring him down here because he forgot something." I gently touched her arm, prompting her to turn towards me. "I interview folks your age every day," I said. "I've heard their stories. Good men and loving husbands who do things totally out of character and don't even remember. That's what delusional thinking does to someone. You start to think or imagine things that aren't true." I hesitated, propping my left foot up on the picnic table bench. "Some even hallucinate. They see and hear things that aren't there. It's dangerous if they start picking up knives or guns."

She stepped back, a terrified look on her face, as if caught between the present and some horrifying point in the past.

"Maggie, please tell me what happened. I just want to help you and John."

"Will you tell the doctor if I tell you?"

"I have to," I said, patting her shoulder. "If you're in danger because of something John doesn't even know he's doing, we can help."

"I'll tell you, but first, let's check on him."

"Fair enough," I said, leading her back through the ambulance entrance to the ER nursing station. I glanced at the chart rack and noticed that his medical chart was missing.

"Where's John Dalton?" I asked the ER unit secretary.

"Radiology."

"Head CT?"

"Yeah."

"What's going on, Michael?" Maggie asked.

"Dr. Halston ordered a test to rule out any kind of hemorrhage or stroke activity. It's standard procedure, nothing out of the ordinary. Let me see what I can find out."

"How long will he be gone?"

"Fifteen or twenty minutes," I said as I led her down the hallway to the grief room. "Go ahead and wait in here. I'll be back in a few minutes."

She nodded, a nervous smile on her forlorn face. "Please hurry back."

"I will."

I hustled back down the hallway to the ER doctors' lounge and knocked on the door. A gruff voice ordered me in. Although surly at times, I liked Dr. Halston. He listened on complicated cases, especially those involving the elderly where it was often difficult to distinguish between medical problems and what might be symptoms of a psychiatric condition. "Dr. Halston, have you seen the 76-year-old male brought in by the police?"

"Working him up," he said, his eyes locked on his computer screen. "I don't expect to find any acute medical problems. What's the game plan?"

"I'm not sure. He's showing signs of dementia but has no prior psych history."

"So what are you telling me?" he asked as he scrolled down his screen.

"It bothers me that the police brought him in," I said. "His wife was close to telling me what happened but she's protecting him."

"What do you think happened?"

"He says he woke up from his nap, thought an intruder was in the house, and ran him out," I said. "My gut tells me he woke up delusional and chased his wife, thinking she was the bad guy. What's strange is how lucid he is now."

He pulled away from his computer screen and turned towards me. "Sounds like psych should admit him for observation, if nothing else."

"He wants to go home and his wife wants the same," I said. "From a risk standpoint, though…"

"Tell you what," he said, turning back towards his keyboard, "call Dr. Baxter and see if he'll come down. He should be around. We've got a medical staff meeting tonight."

"That's fine," I said and headed back to the nursing station to call Dr. Thomas Baxter, III, Faith General's newest psychiatrist and one they paid a fortune to get. He came with an Ivy League background and an ego to match. He was young — forty-two years old — good-looking, witty among his peers, and a total bastard to the blue-collar staff. He was spearheading a major-league drug study for Alzheimer's patients on the hospital's geriatric-psych unit.

I paged Baxter, who chastised me for bothering him until I mentioned that Dr. Halston requested the consult. I slammed the phone down and walked back to update Maggie.

"Does he think something's wrong?" she asked, standing nervously in the doorway.

"He wanted to rule out any medical complications."

"So what happens after that?" she asked as she sat on the front edge of the couch. "Can I take him home? It's getting late and..."

"He wanted a second opinion, so he had me call Dr. Baxter," I said, dreading his involvement for fear his demeaning bedside manner would anger the two of them.

"Who is he?"

"He's the medical director of our geriatric unit upstairs. He's a psychiatrist," I reluctantly added. "He just wants to interview John and ask you a few questions as well."

"But why?" she asked, her voice quivering. "Why a psychiatrist?"

"We're concerned about your safety as well as John's," I said. "You've got to tell me what happened. Please, so I can help."

She motioned for me to shut the assessment office door.

chapter four

"IT STARTED LIKE ANY OTHER day for us," she said, describing in her down-home charming way their daily rituals. From early morning coffee on the back deck to mid-morning strolls in Maggie's rose garden to afternoon walks and John's late afternoon naps on his old recliner while she cooked supper, the pair reveled in their time together.

"He naps about forty-five minutes," she continued. "Did I tell you I've noticed some changes in him? He forgets that he's just done something, or gets stuck trying to get the right words out. He gets frustrated." She looked up, her tired eyes gleaming. "I coerce him out to the back yard. Good ol' sunshine and fresh air work wonders most days. But..." She exhaled slowly.

I waited on her to proceed, all the while enjoying flashbacks of crawling under Mom's rose bush to retrieve many a baseball, sockball, corkball, you name it, we played it in our backyard.

"He can't see all the changes and thinks I'm being overprotective. Maybe I am." She twirled her wedding band around her finger. "Now he'll be the first to tell you that he went to war with our son, Matthew." She leaned back, smiling. "He's fifty-four. Lives in California with his wife. His two daughters, our grandkids, are grown and on their own. Our daughter, Jenny, she's seven years younger than Matthew. She's doing well.

Went through a divorce recently and held her own, much to her Daddy's surprise. He was ready to bring her and her three teenage girls home, but Jenny loves North Carolina. She visits several times a year. Getting John and Matthew together?" She frowned and shrugged her bony shoulders. "They're too much alike. Both gentle as lambs around their women, but bull-headed when it comes to backing down on something they strongly believe in.

"What happened between them?" I asked, the voices in my head screaming to get the goods on what happened, hand the case off and go home.

"Their falling out came years ago when Matthew refused to go to West Point and deemed himself a conscientious objector. John's never forgiven him for that, and Matthew has never felt like what he did was wrong." She hung her head momentarily. "It's sad that father and son can't let go of something that happened so long ago."

"And they haven't spoken since?"

"I've tried to bring them back together." She clasped her fingers and placed them in her lap, her right hand always feeling its way back to her wedding band. "If there's one thing I wish I could change, it's that John let go of his old Army pride and call his son."

I nodded and glanced down at my clipboard, yearning to clock out and head home, yet genuinely intrigued with Maggie and her DiMaggio-like man, not to mention the unexpected flashbacks playing out in my head.

"The bad dreams started about a month ago," she continued. "He'd wake up from his nap confused, sometimes angry, telling others to leave us alone. I'd coax him back, gently talk him down, and he'd tell me it must have been a nightmare, and that was that."

"Did he wake up from a bad dream earlier today?" I asked.

"I didn't hear him get up," she said. "Sometimes I'll turn on my little TV in the kitchen."

28

I nodded and leaned forward, hoping to get to the punch line this go-around.

"I knew something was wrong," she continued. "The way he grabbed me." She clutched the arm of the old couch. "I was afraid to turn around. I thought somebody had broken into the house. Then, he yelled." Maggie shook her head. "Oh, it was an awful sound and so loud, as if it wasn't coming from him. And then I saw the knife…" She hung her head.

"It's okay," I consoled, caught somewhere between my Hollywood persona and genuine empathy. I set my clipboard down and leaned forward on one knee. "It's all right."

She took a deep breath, gathering herself. "I yelled his name, and he let go of me. That's when I ran outside." She shifted to the edge of the couch, fully alert, as if back in the moment. "I thought if I talked to him from a distance, he'd come back to me. He's never…" She went on to describe how her neighbor saw what was happening and called #911.

"But he didn't come after you again with the knife," I said, settling back in my chair.

"No, he just stood by the back deck door yelling, 'Get outta here! Get outta here!' He didn't even put up a fuss when the officers handcuffed him." She shook her head, a pained look on her face. "I hated seeing him led away like that, and from our home. My neighbor wanted to come with me, but I told her everything would be okay. She and her husband know John would never hurt me. I'm sure he'll be fine once I get him back home. He'll be okay, don't you think?"

I nodded and remained silent, wishing I could disappear. Wishing I could make Maggie understand that her beloved husband wasn't returning home with her tonight.

"I just want to take him home. He'll be lost without me. Is he back from those tests?"

chapter five

DRESSED IN HIS TAILORED ATTIRE with a bold blue tie, Doctor Thomas Baxter III arrived looking like he'd strolled off the cover of GQ. He was definitely on top of his game. With a hint of salt and pepper in his slicked-back hair, broad shoulders on his six-foot athletic frame, and a movie star face to go with his baby blue eyes, he was accustomed to turning heads wherever he walked, or drove for that matter. His $100,000 Mercedes turned a few heads as well among the blue-collar hospital clan, some of whom lived in homes worth less than his four-wheel ride or diamond-studded Rolex.

Baxter made no bones about his style and wealth. He wore his thousand-dollar wardrobe and million-dollar smile like royalty. Among his peers, the half-dozen or so other psychiatrists who treated patients at Faith General, Baxter was a godsend. Prior to his heralded arrival four months before, he had practiced in the northeast, developing his reputation as an expert in the field of Alzheimer's research while charming his way up the national research-funding ladder. His wit and wherewithal finally paid off as he arrived at Faith General with a seven-figure drug study neatly packaged in his back pocket.

It was a tremendous financial shot in the arm for a mid-sized hospital struggling to stay afloat in a shark-infested healthcare town. Over the past ten years, Nashville had become an industry giant, home to two of the nation's finest hospitals — St. Thomas, known internationally for its work with heart transplants, and Vanderbilt University Hospital, one of the most prestigious medical schools in the country. In addition, three of the nation's largest healthcare corporations had set up shop in the Music City. For a two-bit player like Faith General to land such a lucrative research deal was quite the coup, whose general was none other than Thomas Baxter, III, MD.

"I'm Dr. Baxter," he said, extending his limp hand to both John and Maggie.

"Who are you?" John fired back.

"He's a specialist," I said. "Dr. Halston, the ER doctor, requested that Dr. Baxter talk to you a few minutes. Is that okay?"

"I'm ready to go home," John growled.

"It's okay, Honey," Maggie said as she stroked his hand. "Just talk to the doctor a minute, and I'm sure we'll be on our way." She looked at me for reassurance. I forced a smile.

"Excuse us," Dr. Baxter said to me. I hesitated for a moment, a brief one at that as he shooed me out like an old dog.

I hustled back to the assessment office, cussing Baxter for his arrogance, yet thankful that he'd provided the out I needed to hand this case off and head home to my booze and TV buttons, to no calls, no responsibilities, and nobody wanting anything from me. That's what I lived for. On this night, however, flashbacks of my parents filled my mind as I typed John's assessment. Vignettes of my elderly parents, along with my son, and countless opportunities to spend time with them lost. And the one thing that I swore I'd never do with my own son — I'd stopped trying to reel him in after my divorce and erected a communication barrier so high that he couldn't climb over it even if he wanted to.

"Quittin' time," David, a long-time co-worker, called out.

"Gettin' there," I said.

"Need me to finish your case?" he asked. "What is it? A geri-psych male?"

I grabbed John's printed assessment. "If you don't mind..." I clipped all of the paperwork and handed it to him. "Baxter saw him in the ER. The patient needs a bed, and check back with Baxter to see if he's going to follow him or pass him off to the on-call doc. Otherwise, just call report. It's straight-up Medicare, no pre-cert needed. That's it."

David frowned. "That's it?"

I playfully threw my hands up in protest. "Have I ever left you a nasty case?"

"You don't wanna go there," he fired back.

"Ok, I gave you the naked schizophrenic last month, but at least she didn't smack you."

He grinned. "I'd forgotten that one."

"How do you forget a three-hundred-pound naked woman?"

"As quickly as possible," he mused.

"I can assure you that other than a 76-year-old-male, who doesn't want to be admitted, and his wife of fifty-six years, who wants to take him home, the case is a breeze."

"The usual, huh?" he said. "Make the doctor out to be the bad guy since he is the one forcing the admission."

"Easy to do with Baxter."

"You owe me."

"Yes, I do." I smiled, patted David on the shoulder, and headed out the side door and down the back hallway towards the time clock, the voices in my head playing ping-pong with my emotions. My mind screamed at me to bolt, insisting there was nothing else I could do with this case. My heart kept seeing my parents and asking if this were them, would I run out now and make them wait another hour or two, much less be told by a total stranger that they had no choice about John being admitted? On top of that, my teammates were already bogged down with complicated cases. Why dump my mess on one of them?

I got to the time clock, grabbed my badge to clock out and stopped in mid-swipe, pounding the wall with my left fist. I returned to the ER looking for Dr. Baxter, but he had already retired to his sixth floor suite. I stopped at the nursing station, only to be told that Dr. Halston was not in the best of moods at the moment. He'd gone from stitching a screaming kid's arm to patching a factory worker's damaged eye. In between, he'd ordered x-rays on two other patients and labs on a 41-year-old, soon-to-be, psych patient from a boarding home. She was singing "How Great Thou Art" one minute and taking swings at anybody within arm's reach the next.

"Get her moved as soon as she clears," Dr. Halston snapped as he grabbed another chart and headed for room three.

I caught him on the run. "Have you talked with Dr. Baxter regarding John Dalton?"

"Check his chart," he barked. "See if he wrote an order."

Back at the nursing station, I grabbed John's chart and tried to read Dr. Baxter's scribbled note but couldn't decipher it. As I turned to find one of the nurses, a document attached to the inside front flap of his chart caught my eye.

"I knew it," I mumbled.

"Knew what?" asked Carol, another co-worker and good friend from the assessment office. She was preparing to take an alcoholic male up to the dual unit.

"Baxter committed my patient to the geri-psych unit."

"What'd you expect?" she said as she gathered the admission

papers. "He needs patients for his Alzheimer's study. Haven't you heard? Whatever he wants, he gets around here."

"Yeah, well…" I smirked. "How am I going to explain this to Maggie?"

"Maggie?" she asked, turning towards me.

"The patient's wife," I said. "They're good people. I hate to see him up on that unit."

"Is that the old guy the police brought in earlier?"

"Yeah."

"I thought he'd attacked his wife."

I turned to face her. "It's not that simple."

"Oh, really?" She placed the medical record back into the ER chart rack.

"What's that supposed to mean?" I fired back.

"It's never bothered you before when some old coot got committed. Why this case?"

I hesitated, still unsure myself. "They're different."

"Different?" She shot me a look. "Is that the best you can come up with?"

"They just don't deserve this, okay?"

She leaned in towards me. "Are you ever going to let that Hollywood façade down long enough to feel something?"

I looked at her and shook my head. Carol could get by chastising me because I liked and respected her work ethic and her way of looking at life. It didn't hurt that she looked mighty fine in her black jeans and boots and Hippie-like shirt sleeves rolled up to her elbows, her brown hair pulled back and tied in a thick pony-tail, her forty-something-year-old face aging gracefully with no sign or need for anything plastic. She looked like the painter / artist she longed to be, and was, when not hustling psych admissions with me at work.

"What did Halston say?" she asked.

"He's the one who told me to call Baxter."

"Hope he hasn't sold out like everyone else around here."

I held up a copy of the involuntary committal form. "How do I explain this?"

"Maybe Baxter did."

"Yeah, right," I sneered. "No telling what he told them. Guess I'm fixing to find out."

"Sooner than you think," Carol said, motioning me to turn around.

Housekeeping, mop bucket and all, had forgotten to check behind them again, allowing John and Maggie the brief but well-timed opportunity to slip out of the locked doors. "Maggie?" I hustled over to them. "What's going on?"

"I'm taking my husband and we're leaving," she replied as she grabbed hold of John's hand and pulled him down the ER hall.

"What did Dr. Baxter say?" I asked, matching their every step.

"That he wanted him to stay in the hospital for a few days," she said, "up on some unit for crazy old people. I told him John wasn't staying."

I finally managed to get in front of them. "So what did he say when you told him no?" I asked, gently blocking their path.

"Something about keeping him here anyway, that John was a danger, and as a physician he couldn't let him go."

"And?" I managed to coax them into one of the ER assessment rooms, all the while trying to get security Pete's attention. "Did Dr. Baxter explain what he meant when he said he couldn't let John leave?"

"I guess he did, I don't know," Maggie said, clearly disgusted. "He was talking so fast and..." She looked up at me, her eyes begging me to let them go. "We just want to go home, Michael. Is there a law against that?"

"Yeah, let's go home," John snapped. "Are you going stop us from leaving?"

I eased forward, facing John. "Don't you think it would be in your best interest to stay in the hospital tonight? Let the doctors look at you and maybe prescribe some medicine to help with those bad dreams?"

"I'm fine now," he said. "Maggie can take care of me. I'm not staying. C'mon Honey." He grabbed her hand and started towards the door.

I casually blocked them again, hoping to calm him down. "Maggie, help me here," I pleaded. "The doctor has the authority to commit someone to stay against his will if he feels that the patient is at risk to harm himself or someone else." I reached over and patted John's shoulder. "I'm sorry things have happened this way, but we have no choice. He has to stay at least through tonight."

"You told me we could go home earlier," she said. "Leaving him here is no help. He'll be lost without me."

"I'm not so sure I agree with the doctor," I said, slowly redirecting them back into the room and into chairs, "but I can't override Dr. Baxter's decision." I eased the door shut and leaned against it. "And frankly, if I'm in the doctor's shoes," I turned my gaze towards Maggie, "I'd have no choice but to commit John. He went after you with a knife. We know that he wasn't aware of what he was doing, but that's the point." I kneeled down on one knee, looking up at them. "Who's to say he won't do it again tomorrow, or the next day? It's in his best interest to be admitted for observation and evaluation. Maybe the doctor can find a medication that will help." I leaned in closer to them. "I hate that this is happening, but we want the two of you safe." I looked over at Maggie. "Returning home tonight is not safe."

I stood and gently touched John's shoulder. "It's not as bad as you think on the unit," I said. "There's nurses and techs 'round the clock, and the doctor will see you again in the morning. All we want to do is get you to feeling better. Help clear those cobwebs and get you back home to Maggie."

"How long will he have to stay?" she asked, agonized.

"It depends on how he's doing. Could be a week, or just a few days if he's responding well."

"Can I stay with him?"

I hated answering that question. Like most people, she had no idea that we were placing her spouse on a locked geriatric psychiatric unit. Although a full service hospital with a variety of medical units, on any given day over half of Faith General's beds were filled with psychiatric patients. In years gone by, psychiatry had been the golden goose for the hospital. However with the onset of managed care, the only way the hospital stayed afloat on psych patients was to "run volume and run it lean" as the ivory tower bean counters denied ever saying. The end result on all six psych units, each with a maximum of 20 beds, was that programs stayed full most of the time, yet had far too few staff to maintain the peace. Without question, the most difficult unit to work on was the geri-psych unit.

I turned to face her. "They don't have accommodations on the unit or in the hospital for family."

"What am I...?" She hung her head but only for a moment. She turned and looked at her man sitting quietly, a dazed look on his face. "Honey, they want you to stay in the hospital tonight. I don't want you to, but they're telling me you have to stay."

"Who's telling you that?" he snapped.

"The doctor, Dr. Baxter. He feels like you need to be checked out for a night or two."

"I'm not staying! You hear me, Maggie. Please take me home."

"Honey, please don't. I can't go against the doctor's order. I..." Tears welled up in her eyes as she stroked John's troubled face.

"Let me get everything lined up," I said. "That way we can get you up to the unit and Maggie can go with you. You'll be able to ask the staff questions about the program." I knew that the longer he had in the ER to brood, or see Maggie sullen and tearful, the worse things could get. I looked at Maggie, hoping to gain some measure of support. "Can you stay here while I finish up? It'll take about twenty minutes."

Maggie nodded as she held his hand, her forlorn face a far cry from the vibrant woman sharing their story earlier. I patted both she and John one last time, relieved that my ER psychiatric watch for the day could finally end, yet saddened that neither knew what awaited them on the geri-psych unit known as Passages.

chapter six

I HUNG THE OFFICE PHONE UP and glanced at the wall clock. It was seven-thirty. "Where is he?" I muttered, referring to Greg, our 7p to 7a graveyard shift worker.

"Something about a tractor-trailer jackknifing," Carol said as she smacked our bipolar fax machine and emphatically poked the numbers on its faded façade.

"Not tonight," I moaned. "How late?"

"'Bout an hour," she said. "I thought you'd left."

"I did." I slumped down in my chair as David breezed in.

"He's on his period again David," Carol teased.

"I thought he was last week," he chimed in as he filled her coffee cup.

I shook my head in disgust.

"Look on the bright side," she said.

"Can't wait to hear it," I muttered.

"You get to spend more quality time with the old couple who touched you."

"Oh my god," David said, "is the old man going soft on us?" He turned towards me. "You came back to pick up the case that you gave me?" He reached out and grabbed Carol's arm. "Check his pulse. He must be hallucinating."

"Command hallucinations," I said with a blank stare as they sipped their coffee. "To poison my co-workers." I walked out, amused for the moment, but determined to complete John's case and head home. I grabbed the remainder of his ER paperwork at the nursing station and approached John and Maggie for the long walk up to Passages, Faith General's 20-bed, lock-down, geriatric, psychiatric unit.

Maggie saw me coming and cringed. I knew that if I gave her any opportunity to stall or barter we might never make it up to the unit. "Okay, let's head upstairs so that we can get you settled in," I said to John as I nodded to Maggie. She acknowledged my cue, nudging John to start the slow procession down the hallway to the elevators.

We inched along at a snail's pace, John and Maggie arm-in-arm the entire way, with me meandering alongside them, praying that John did not have another delusional moment. We eased onto the elevator for the ride up to the second floor.

We rounded the corner and started down the last hallway leading to the unit. As we strolled past the stairwell door and several offices, Maggie suddenly stopped, a terrified look distorting her face. I knew what had just happened — I had seen the elopement risk sign on the door too. I hated those signs. Even tried to tell the white collars that the signs were frightening to folks just coming onto the floor. They agreed but never bothered to spend the extra few bucks for less obtrusive signs. Granted, housekeeping, food services and others entering the locked unit needed to be cautious and not let a patient slip out the door. But to hang a large, bright red, ELOPEMENT RISK sign on the outside of the door was disheartening to family members and downright demoralizing to new patients and loved ones like John and Maggie.

"It's okay." I urged them onward. "That's just to remind

housekeeping and cafeteria staff. We wouldn't want someone to wander out and get lost."

John took three steps and stopped, looking directly at me. "Maggie said you would help us. What gives you the right to lock me up in this place?"

I turned to Maggie for support, but she was having second thoughts. I prompted them onward, edging ever closer to the entrance. She held him tight as they teetered towards the locked double doors.

"Can I stay with him awhile?" she asked.

"I'm sure the staff will want to talk with you."

John stopped again and turned towards Maggie. "Why are they making me stay? Can't you take me home?"

"Honey, it's just for a night or two to help get your medications regulated. You said that blood pressure medication was making you too tired."

I keyed the electronic lock on the wall next to the steel-door entrance, hoping to minimize the often times frightening feeling of locked doors, while at the same time praying that the unit was not in shambles. Escorting new admits onto any of Faith General's six psychiatric units had inherit risks, however geri-psych brought into play pitfalls that challenged all of staff's senses.

"You ready?" I asked, prompting them to go in.

"I don't like this," John muttered as he entered the unit, Maggie right beside him, clutching his arm all the way.

"Oh my…" She stopped.

I secured the door and turned back to lead them down the hall when we were confronted by an elderly woman.

"Believe in the works of the Lord," the old woman demanded. "Repent and be saved!" she cried, stretching her diminutive frame as tall as she could in hopes of making eye contact with John. "Serpent, be healed!" she yelled at him and scampered down the hallway in slow motion, her flowered gown flapping in the breeze of a hallway fan strategically placed to subdue a sickening odor seeping from one of the bedrooms.

"It's okay," I said as I patted John on the back, hoping to ease him down to the nursing station where I could drop them off and be on my merry way.

Neither one moved, both dumbfounded by the unit's welcome wagon. It didn't help matters that the unit was down one staff member and the nurses were late getting out of their shift change report. The hallway was a frightening mess as several patients wandered about, lost in a mumbling daze while one overworked and underpaid nurse's tech cleaned up the debris left in the dining room.

"The nursing station is this way," I said, edging them forward, hoping we'd make it without further incident. We inched onward, past the brightly lit, recently remodeled dayroom where a big screen TV was blaring. Two elderly men sat stone-faced, neither aware of our presence.

"That's a nice TV," Maggie said, patting John's hand. "See, it's not as bad as you think."

We crept by the next room where two women laid in their respective beds, both staring at the ceiling, oblivious to the procession peering at them.

We moved beyond the bed-ridden pair to the next room where an old man sat on the edge of his bed muttering and masturbating. Embarrassed, I urged John and Maggie onward.

We finally made it to the nursing station, but not before one final plea from the church lady to, "Repent or be cast into hell with all the other sorry souls of this earth!" I'd hoped to put John in one of the chairs across from the nursing station, however all three were occupied with patients waiting for their medications. All three looked like they were long overdue as one rocked obsessively, one stared blankly into space, and the third one, God bless him, was a 92-year-old man I'd admitted several days earlier by the name of Robert. He was a retired railroad engineer on his fifth stay in the Passages program in the past ten months. Seems his nursing home couldn't contain his sudden urges to crawl into bed with the nearest female resident he could find.

"Hello Robert? Remember me?" I reached over to shake his hand and then thought better of the idea. He motioned me to move closer.

"Got any Viagra?" he whispered.

"For what?" I whispered back, making sure no one heard me.

"See that nurse over there. I'd..."

I didn't give him a chance to finish, stepping quickly to the counter. "Excuse me." I smiled at the nurse. "I've got John, our new admission, and his wife, Maggie. Can we..."

"You'll have to wait for the evening nurse," she snapped, never bothering to look up. "I ain't about to start another admission this late. Why didn't you call and let us know you was comin'?"

"I called report," I said, trying to sound professional but angered at her lack of common sense courtesy.

"Michael, can I talk to you a minute?" Maggie asked.

"Sure." I led her several feet away while John stood motionless at the nursing station, dazed by all that was happening around him.

"This place," her voice cracked, "these people..." Her hand trembled as she motioned towards John. "My John doesn't belong up here. This looks more like a nursing home than a hospital. He doesn't need this. He needs to be home with me."

"I wish I could tell you to take him home," I said, "but I can't. He has to stay at least one night until Dr. Baxter sees him again in the morning."

"I don't like that man," she whispered, "and sure don't trust him. Can we request another doctor?"

"You can," I said, glancing at John, "but give Dr. Baxter the benefit of the doubt for now. If I call another doctor tonight, he's not going to let him leave until he sees him in the morning."

She leaned into me. "It's just not right!" she emphatically stated in my ear.

"I know your first impression's not been good," I said, reaching over to touch her left arm, "but give it a chance. They do good work up here. I've seen patients when they leave, and some are doing much better." I pulled back from her. "Give it a chance to work." I waited on her to look me in the eye. "Don't forget — John went after you with a knife earlier today."

"In all our years, he's never so much as laid a hand on me."

"I hesitate to share this with you," I said as I glanced around, edging closer to her while watching John to make sure he was okay. "There's a man on this unit as we speak."

"What man?"

"A patient I admitted last week. He accidentally shot his wife of forty-seven years. Thought she was sneaking men into her bedroom at night. He thinks he killed one of those men. Still believes it. He had no history of violence and a wonderful marriage until his delusions took over."

"But John would never..."

"When he's thinking clearly, of course he wouldn't," I said. "But look at what happened earlier. And who's to say it won't happen again? Only, the next time you might not get away. It's worth a few nights in this program, no matter what you think of it at this point, to see if Dr. Baxter can find a medication that will help. Trust me, I'm not crazy about his bedside manner, but he's well respected nationally for his work with the elderly. And right now, John deserves the best we can offer when it comes to finding something that will hopefully eliminate his delusions.

Please, give it a chance to work. I'll be around the next couple of days. I'll check in on him."

"Would you please do that for me?"

"I'll be glad to." I replied, patting her on the shoulder. "Now, how 'bout we stir these nurses up so John can get settled in."

John smiled as she caressed his hand, assuring him that everything would be okay.

The church lady made rounds again, assuring one and all that the end was near.

The end, however, was nowhere in sight for John and Maggie Dalton.

chapter seven

"Thought you'd left," said David, leaning back in his chair.

I plopped down next to him as Carol walked in. "Just unwinding before I head out," I said, checking the front zipper of my weathered backpack.

"You unwinding with us?" Carol teased.

I smirked as I stashed my belongings – chap stick, gum, pen, eye drops, and a small, frayed, batch of three-by-five cards stapled together, condensing a multitude of contacts, codes, and cunning shortcuts to manipulate the system and keep patients moving through the often times, murky, mental health maze.

"You feel okay old man?" she pestered, peering at me with her arms folded.

"Fine," I snapped, turning back towards David.

"Excuse me." She sat down at the third computer station, the one facing away from the hallway where two bipolar patients swiveled their heads between watching Judge Judy on the boob tube and staring at us, the half-wall-to-ceiling Plexiglas providing patients and staff ample opportunity to study each other's every move.

I rolled my shabby chair towards Carol. "Hey…" I waited

patiently, hoping she would turn back towards me. She obliged, but not before making me wait long enough to let me know that I'd hurt her feelings. "I'm sorry," I said. "I just..."

She turned around to face me. "What?"

"Life's cruel sometimes." I eased my chair back, unaccustomed to sharing personal feelings with anyone, much less an attractive female. "Here's a couple totally committed to each other for fifty-six years, truly in love and enjoying life. Seeing that spark in their eyes when she stroked his face..." I hesitated, head down momentarily for fear of showing emotion. I looked up and continued. "Then boom! You're standing in the kitchen one day and the love of your life has a knife to your throat. How do you deal with that?" I slowly retreated to the safety of my work space.

"He's got Alzheimer's?" David asked, stepping over to the printer to pick up referral information on another patient.

"Who knows?" I set my backpack down on the floor. "His wife reported increased memory loss and confusion, especially when he wakes up from his afternoon nap. That's what happened today. He woke up and thought she was an intruder."

"That's scary," Carol said, pulling back from her keyboard. "Does she feel safe with him at home?"

"Home sure smells better than the alternative," I said, glancing at my computer screen. "Have you been up there lately?"

"I took a patient up earlier," she said. "Why?"

"I was embarrassed," I said. "It was bad enough just getting to the nursing station, and then to have staff run their mouths right in front of the family."

"I get that all the time," David chimed in. "They complain if census drops and staff's sent home, yet the minute we start filling 'em back up, they bitch about having to work and don't think twice about doing it in front of the patient."

"Who's the little lady hell-bent on saving everyone?" I asked.

"Ah, the church lady." Carol laughed. "I admitted her last week. She's harmless."

"We see it every day, but Maggie and John have never been exposed to a locked unit filled with crazy old people running around yelling, 'Repent and be saved you devils!' "

"She'd take him home tonight?" Carol asked.

"In a heartbeat."

"So why doesn't she?" asked David.

"Baxter," I said.

"He committed him?"

"Of course," Carol snapped. "He needs patients for his research study."

"Would you have let him walk?" David asked me.

"I don't know." I slowly stood, glancing about the office. "Without Maggie's determined consent? Absolutely not. I'd commit him in a heartbeat." I signed out of the computer. "Even with Maggie accepting responsibility, it's not tonight I worry about so much as tomorrow afternoon when he wakes up from his nap."

"Yeah, but like we've always said," Carol grabbed the newest referral off the printer, "you can't keep people locked up because of what might happen. And you sure shouldn't be admitting them to turn them into research guinea pigs."

I hurled my backpack over my left shoulder. "Money talks," I said, "and Baxter's loaded."

"He treats us like dirt," Carol said as she slid over to our referral board. "I hate when he's on call. What a jerk on the phone."

"But, does he know what he's doing?" David questioned. "Is he a good doctor?"

"He's supposedly one of the best at treating Alzheimer's." I pushed my chair up against the counter. "But then again, who knows? Remember when they said Dr. Kaskin was world renowned with schizophrenics? That guy was certifiably crazy!"

"What happened to him?" David asked.

"He bolted back to Vanderbilt," I said. "Didn't care much for us blue collar folk on the poor side of town."

Carol handed me my Pepsi. "Then why would Baxter, an Ivy League doc with all that money and prestige, wind up here? Why not Vanderbilt, or St. Thomas?"

"Guess we'll find out, huh? See ya."

I eased the office door shut and slid out the side door entrance, my psychiatric tour-of-duty done for the day.

⤳

"What are you doing?" Carol hollered down the ER hallway.

"I'm the one with Alzheimer's," I joked. "Got to my car and didn't have my keys."

"You sure you can take care of yourself old man?" she teased, a seductive smile at that.

"That's debatable." I waved and scurried back to the office.

"Michael," David said, "I just told the geri-psych unit you were gone."

"What'd they want?"

"The wife of that patient wanted to talk to you again."

I grabbed my keys from the cubicle drawer and reached for the phone.

"Let it go, man," he said. "I told 'em you were gone. There's nothing else you can do at this point. Get out of here while you can."

"I think I will," I said, surveying the hallway. "This hasn't been a fun day."

"No, and you know the rest of the week will be wild with the census down."

"Oh, man, you know what else?" I stashed my keys in my pocket.

He turned and glanced at another psych patient the ER nurse and security had just escorted back, a straggly-haired, middle-aged, homeless-looking male toting his tattered guitar case and three garbage bags. "Must be a full moon," David mused.

"The house will be rockin," I mumbled as I slid out the back door, officially ending my twelve-hour day. In addition to John's case, I'd assessed a 21-year-old status post overdose who was flunking out of college and too ashamed to tell his highly successful parents, two bipolar females, both off their medications and extremely manic, one schizophrenic male threatening to take my head off at any point during the interview, one frequent-flyer male with AIDS threatening to infect me and everyone else in ER if we didn't admit him, and one obnoxious drunk, another of our frequent flyers, who knew the two magic words for admission. "I'm suicidal" was an instant winner, even though this same drunk had told me the same story and plan of suicide only two months earlier. He had no intentions of harming himself. I knew it. He knew it. But the hospital had no choice from a liability standpoint. And the truth of the matter was we never did know what might happen if we called their bluff and discharged them back to the streets.

Two months ago, a frequent flyer told me he was suicidal and then changed his mind after I'd made all the arrangements to admit him. I got him to sign a safety contract and convinced the ER doc to let him walk since the guy had never actually attempted suicide. We got word two weeks later that he'd killed himself — slashed himself real good with a box cutter and died in a lowdown motel in the Music City's, drug-infested, red light district.

I hustled across the parking lot towards my car.

"Michael?"

I recognized that feeble voice. Oh, how I wanted to jump in my car and scramble to the safety of my apartment where I could shut out the world. On any other night, I would have done just that — ignored it and gone my way.

"Maggie? Is that you?" I turned around.

"Michael, I'm sorry to bother you again. I know you must be tired."

"I'm okay," I lied, walking over to her. "How about you? Did you get John settled in?"

"No..." She hung her head momentarily. "He feels like I abandoned him."

"I'm so sorry."

She looked up at me, those motherly eyes deadened with sadness. "He just looked so lost."

I reached out and touched her shoulder, wishing I could take her pain and anguish away. As much as my heart went out to John, she didn't deserve this fate either. Fifty-six years of love and loyalty to her man was not supposed to be rewarded like this.

I longed to tell her good night, good luck, and head to the house. But...

For the first time in what seemed like months, the stirring in my soul was not associated with pain and rejection. It was a warm feeling that I hadn't felt in a long, long time — genuine empathy for another human being, not the Hollywood version twenty-five years in the mental health trenches had taught me.

"How 'bout I follow you home," I blurted out.

"Oh no," Maggie said, a warm smile on her face, "it's quite a ways."

"I bet John's like most guys," I said. "Heaven forbid we let a woman drive us around."

She nodded. "John does prefer to do the driving. But, you don't have to..."

"I'd be honored to escort you home. And besides," I stepped closer to her, "I'd sleep better knowing you made it home safe. Where's your car?"

"It's in the lower lot."

"I won't take no for an answer," I replied, opening my car door. "Here." I reached out to her. "Get in and I'll drive you around."

"You don't have to do this, Michael."

"I know."

She was right. I didn't have to do this. Yet, it was reassuring to know that I could do something for someone without expecting anything in return. That caring, nurturing, emotionally sensitive side of me had all but died following the events that paralyzed me prior to moving to Nashville eighteen months earlier. Losing my job via a corporate downsizing had demoralized me. Losing my wife of twenty-three years to another man had all but destroyed my sense of self-worth. Yet, neither of those traumatic events plunged me as deep into the abyss as having had my 21-year-old son, my only child, disown me, accusing me of caring more for my work than my own flesh and blood child. His parting shot to me — "Call me when you're ready to be a real father." I shut down emotionally. For weeks on end I couldn't muster the courage to crawl out of my pity pot. Couldn't find a job worthy of my class, but managed to locate a boatload of worthy bars. Worst of all, I lost my Mom's faith in me as a good and decent human being, and became, for a period of time, the one thing that I always swore I'd never become – a lonely bitter man.

The voice in my head countered. *The last thing you need to do is get involved with some old couple, especially off the clock. This can only lead to headaches and trouble.*

"I'll take my chances," I mumbled as I helped Maggie into her car.

"Excuse me?"

"Oh, it was nothing. Now, I'm going to follow you, so don't run off and leave me."

"I can't tell you how much I appreciate…"

Hey idiot! Don't you remember? No contact with patients or their families outside of work. You can't afford to lose this job! It took you long enough to find one.

"Be careful, Maggie."

chapter eight

"BET YOU DIDN'T REALIZE WE were this far out in the country," Maggie said.

I stood in the driveway gazing up at the sky. "I haven't seen this many stars since I was a kid."

"Hurry up now," she said, grabbing my arm. "There's plenty of time to do that on the back porch." She led me up to the front door. "Now where are my keys?"

"Ah yes, keys." I held the storm door open, lost somewhere between lying on my couch and loving my sudden surge of spontaneous humanity.

"Now then." Maggie flipped the living room lights on and locked the front door. "Let me call my neighbor to let her know I'm home and then you can be on your way. I know you must be tired."

"Yes ma'am," I nodded, "it's been a long day." I smiled.

"I'll be right back," Maggie said as she started into the living room. "Make yourself at home. Our phone is out in the den."

I wandered into their living room, a small, formal, seating area with antique tidbits scattered about. From the looks of it, they rarely used the room; the throw pillows on the couch, along with the pictures and trinkets on the coffee table and matching end tables, even the corner bookshelf filled to the ceiling with books and momentous, was flawless.

"Quite a collection, huh?" she said.

I jumped, like a child caught in the cookie jar.

"I didn't mean to startle you."

"That's okay," I said.

Maggie joined me by the bookshelf. "John loves to read. How he savors a good book."

"Has he read all of these?" I asked as I scanned the shelves, spotting an array of old hardbacks.

"Most of them," she said, "several more than once."

"Does he have a favorite?"

Her eyes scanned the shelves. "He told me once that the greatest gift he ever received was an old diary." She gently pulled a tattered notebook down. "His favorite uncle gave it to him. John used to tell me how it changed his life. As a fifteen-year-old boy who'd already quit school to help support his family, his uncle's inspiring words gave John the courage to dream of a better life."

"That's one dream he definitely fulfilled," I said.

"Many times over, Michael," she said. "Many times over." She stood silent for a moment, gazing at the old diary in her hands, before placing it back on the shelf. "Let me show you one other thing, his most prized possession. Have you got a minute? I know you need to go."

"Sure." I followed her through a formal dining room, complete with cherry table and chairs, and into a large, comfortable den. A quaint, country kitchen was off to the right with an eat-in counter and bar stools separating the two rooms. "This is nice."

"This is home back here," she said. "Here in the den or out on the back deck is where we spend most of our time. John catnaps over there on his recliner. He loves that old chair."

I nodded and smiled, flashbacks of Pop lounging in his old

recliner, the two of us watching a baseball game on the TV while Mom cooked in the kitchen.

"Over here." She directed me to an even larger set of built-in bookcases. "Let's see..." She perused the shelves. "Ah, there it is!" She handed it to me as if it was a live grenade.

I cradled it in my hands. "I haven't held one of these." I held it up close to my eyes, studying the signature on the alum-tanned Holstein cowhide. "I should have known."

"An old Army friend sent it to him as a wedding gift."

"That must have been some friend," I said, staring at the autographed baseball.

"He was the last close friend that John had from the Army."

"I saw clips of Joe DiMaggio on ESPN," I said. "I never knew how great a ballplayer he was. Such grace on the field." I slowly turned the baseball in my hands, my fingers tickling the seams, igniting joyous childhood memories. "They talked about how he was the last of a dying breed of heroes; that the past couple of generations had no idea what an impact the Yankee Clipper had on so many Americans, not just baseball fans." I looked up at Maggie and smiled. "He was a class act."

She nodded. "That he was."

My gaze returned one last time to the baseball. "I better get on down the road," I said, gingerly placing it back on its perch. "I have to be back at the hospital early."

"I'm sorry. I didn't mean to keep you."

"Oh no." I instinctively stepped towards her. "I'm honored that you shared something so special to John. My father would have..." I glanced down at my feet, my mouth scratchy dry, thoughts of how much Pop respected and admired genuine class and humility in any man, but especially DiMaggio. On deck, the voice in my head blasted me again. *Some old woman shows you a fancy baseball and you get emotional? Wake up! You start taking these patients home with you, and you're dead meat. You hear me!* I looked up, took a deep breath and offered Maggie a warm smile.

"Well, the least I can do is send you home with supper," she said, hustling into the kitchen.

"That's okay, I'm fine. I've got..." I eased over to the kitchen counter as Maggie retrieved several bowls from her refrigerator. "Had this ready for supper tonight." Maggie hesitated, a forlorn look on her face. She quickly gathered herself and set a roast pan out on the counter. "I've got an old microwave plate here somewhere. You do have a microwave don't you."

"Couldn't live without it," I said, my taste buds drifting back to Mom's Sunday best, a far cry from the three-day-old pizza at home.

"You like roast beef?"

"Yes ma'am," I replied, unable to recall the last time I'd had a home-cooked meal.

"Well, there's no sense in letting this roast and green beans go bad, now is there?"

I wasn't about to argue with her, especially after she whipped out the creamed potatoes and gravy, corn-on-the-cob, and threw in a homegrown tomato.

"Now that should feed you for the night," she said as she handed me the food neatly packaged in a paper sack. "Michael, I'm grateful. I don't know what I would have done without you."

"No, Maggie," I said, clutching the sack, "I'm the one who needs to say thanks." I had no way of telling her what this night had brought me – rejuvenated feelings of genuine compassion, along with rekindled childhood memories.

"Will you keep an eye on him for me?" she asked. She had a look of fear in her eyes.

I nodded, patted her on the shoulder and headed out into the darkness.

chapter nine

"AM I GLAD TO SEE you," I said to Carol. She set her belongings on the back counter. "Been a bad morning?"

"Two uninsured junkies and Elvis."

"Elvis?"

"Hails from Vegas," I turned towards her, "or so he says." I grabbed Elvis' valuables baggie and held it up for Carol to see. "We have twelve gaudy rings, five gold necklaces, four costume jewelry bracelets, two fake diamond-studded watches, and..." I set the bag down and leaned back in my chair, enjoying her stylish backside in blue jeans. Carol was an attractive woman from my generation. She, too, was divorced and disillusioned about life and relationships. Her two kids were grown and living out-of-state and her parents were deceased. She was easy to talk to, something I seldom encountered with women, or men for that matter. I was more comfortable conversing with Elvis than I was with the vast majority of sane souls I'd come in contact with over the past few years. Carol, though, was different.

She turned from the coffee maker. "And what?"

"And a sole-flapping pair of faded blue-suede shoes," I said with a grin.

"You're joking?"

"Kid you not," I said. "Had 'em wrapped in old tissue paper in his raggedly suitcase. Said he and his wife of twenty-seven years traveled around the country working and performing in small clubs and carnies." I sat up in my chair. "No prior psych history," I said, "no outpatient counseling, no depression, nothing. And then one day last week…" I held my Styrofoam cup out.

She obliged, double sugar included. "What happened?"

"His wife, his goddess as he called her…" I held the cup to my face, inhaled the rich coffee smell, and took a sip. "She died in her sleep," I continued, "lying right next to him in their 1984 Airstream. It was their wedding present to each other and the only home they ever knew." I set my cup down on the counter. "He can't recall the name of the town in Ohio where she died," I said, "but he *knows* how many hairs she had on her head."

"So he has one too many," she said, "winds up in an ER drunk and babbling about wishing he could join his wife, and some 'I-don't-have-time-for-this' ER doc commits him."

"And he gets here," I said, "and of all the ER docs to be on early this morning."

"Thompson," Carol muttered.

"Yep. He doesn't care what I think, even though I've spent forty minutes with Elvis and *know* he's not suicidal." I turned back towards my keyboard. "He was drunk! The last thing we need to do is slam him upstairs against his will."

"Which doc admitted him?" she asked.

"Matthews."

"Thank God," she said, sitting co-pilot with me, her stylish brown hair hanging freely below her shoulders.

"That's what I told the poor guy, that Dr. Matthews would listen and work with him."

"What's he gonna do when he's discharged?"

"The carny life is all he knows," I said, rotating to face her. "It was sad. He said he'd given up on finding, 'the one woman God intended me to be with,' as he put it. He was thirty-four when they met. She was thirty-eight. Both of 'em runaways at seventeen. Neither *ever* looked back." I turned back to my work station.

"Quite the love story," Carol said, "and life they lived."

I slowly turned her way, unable to meet her eyes. "They knew real joy. Elvis and his goddess." I retreated to the solitude and safety of my computer screen.

"I think David is right," she said.

"About?" I asked, my eyes never leaving my computer screen where I tracked patients coming into our ER, always curious as to who might meander through our doors.

"Another case that touched your heart," Carol teased. "Maybe you are getting soft."

I exited the ER screen. "You guys act like I'm some cold-hearted asshole."

"You said it," she teased, a playful smile on her face.

"Why are you so happy this morning?" I snapped. "You find yourself a good man?"

"As a matter of fact..." She held her coy grin.

"What?" I cried. "You want a drum roll?" I leaned towards her and rat-tat-tapped the Formica countertop.

"No..."

"No what?" I stood and stuffed a wad of papers in the recycle bin sitting off to my left. "You don't want a drum roll, or you didn't find a man?"

"No to both," she said, waiting on me to face her.

I obliged, clutching the back of my chair.

"Why are you so concerned?"

"Just looking out for a friend," I said.

"Didn't know you considered me such a good friend," Carol said, easing closer.

I pulled back, a little embarrassed. "Well, I do."

"You're blushing old man."

I plopped back down in my chair, wishing she'd stop calling me old man. "Good to know the blood's still circulating," I said. "Speaking of which, we got a drunk in twelve and a fiery 75-year-old woman out in the ER."

She grabbed a clipboard. "Right up your alley," she quipped.

"What? The drunk?"

"The old lady," she said. "You like older women don't you?"

"You're on a roll this morning," I said, relaxed that our conversation had turned back to business and bantering.

"I just enjoy working with you, that's all," she replied.

That's all?" I fired back without thinking.

"You're blushing again."

"You take the drunk and I'll take the gyrating granny," I said.

She shook her head. "I knew it."

"If granny's admitted, it gives me an excuse to check on John," I said, easing out of my chair. "I'd hoped to sneak up there early this morning. Maggie's probably fit to be tied."

"Another older woman. How many you got?"

"Only one that I'm truly concerned about," I said, stretching one last time before grabbing an assessment packet.

"That old couple really touched you."

"I'll tell you about it later," I said.

"Maybe we'll get a break in the action," she said, brushing by me as she started out the office door. "Anything I need to know about the drunk?"

"He's been here since midnight, and we've never seen him before. Have fun!"

"You too, old man," she said, stepping across the hall and into the drunken man's domain, putrid smell and all.

As I started out the office door, the phone rang. It was Maggie.

"Michael, nobody up there will talk to me. They keep telling me I need a code number or something before they'll even acknowledge that he's there."

"They didn't give you the code number last night?" I asked, watching Carol on our office monitor.

"What code number?"

"Patients are assigned four-digit privacy-code numbers. Family members are notified once the patient decides who can be on the list of approved people."

"Approved people?" she asked, her voice cracking.

"Let me find out what's going on."

"Would you, please?"

"I got one more patient to see, then, I'll go see him."

"You don't think something's happened to him do you? Those nurses were so rude."

"I'm sure he's fine," I said. "I'll call as soon as I can."

"Thanks, Michael."

"No problem. Did you sleep okay last night?"

"Not really. I talked to Matthew, our son in San Francisco, for almost an hour. It was so good to hear from him."

I assured Maggie that I would call her back and started out the door when the phone rang again. It was the ER nurse.

"When are you coming to assess this geriatric patient? We can't..."

"On my way," I snapped. I hustled down the hallway, glancing in each treatment room, wondering where my 75-year-old woman might be. It didn't take long to find her.

"About time ya got here," she cried out. "Where ya been all my life?"

It was all I could do to keep a straight face as Wilma Johnson, AKA WiLou, was indeed gyrating, grinning down at me from high atop her desktop throne. In a flash, she hurled her string-bean body right at me, howling for joy. "I'm all yours, Sonny."

I unraveled the two of us and placed her in a chair as a dumbfounded lab tech stared from the hallway, wondering why a 75-year-old patient had her arms and legs wrapped around me.

"Now what'd you say your name is?" I asked.

"I go by WiLou," she said, standing up, "but for you, I'll go by any ol' name you call me. Come over here and..." She lunged towards me.

I eased her back down, this time sternly addressing her. "Now WiLou, if you can't talk to me right, I'll just have to get one of them mean ol' nurses in here to set you straight. I don't want to do that, but if I can't get some information from you, my boss will think I can't do my job."

She leaned back momentarily and then scooted up to the front of her chair. "What'd you wanna know, Sonny?" she asked, unable to sit still, her legs constantly crossing or foot perpetually tapping the floor.

"How'd you get here?" I asked, relieved that WiLou appeared to be a slam dunk admission to geri-psych.

She dropped her chin and looked up at me with those beady eyes. "Ambulance brung me here."

I sat on top of the desk. "And where do you live?"

"In that nasty ol' nursing home." She uncrossed her legs, her boney fingers repeatedly scratching her nappy head. "Can you get me outta there?"

"Why do you wanna leave?"

"They're mean to me," she pleaded, wringing her hands.

I set my clipboard on the desk and folded my arms, stroking my chin. "What happened this morning that got you sent here?"

"Ah now, do I have to tell ya?" she asked, grinning from ear to ear, revealing a wad of Skoal stuffed in her lower lip.

I had to ask. "Where'd you get that there chaw?"

"What chaw?" She smiled again, juice oozing down her chin.

I smiled back at her. "Don't you ever spit?"

"Naw, I just swallow the juice. Good for your innards."

I felt the rumbling in my gut, warning me to expedite the interview, otherwise she'd be spewing more tobacco juice and I'd be wearing my coffee and Twinkies.

"So why'd they send you here?" I asked again.

"I got mad and threw my breakfast tray at them people."

"Them people?"

"They're poisoning my food!" she cried, leaping up and prancing around the room, carrying on a private conversation with, "those demons" as she shouted to the rooftops. I slipped out the door while she had her back turned. With security finally watching her, I went back to the assessment office to get her admitted.

Carol entered moments later. "How does it feel?"

"How's what feel?" I asked, playfully looking her up and down as she sat next to me.

"To be wanted by 75-year-old women," she mocked. "Must make you feel manly, huh?"

"Actually, it's the best..." I grinned. "No, I'm not going there."

"Chicken."

"Yeah, well, I'll broach this subject with you at a later time," I hinted.

"I'll hold you to that."

Thirty minutes later, I waltzed up to geri-psych with WyLou under my arm, eager to hand her off to the unit staff so that I could check on John. There's nothing like riding a packed elevator with a 75-year-old manic woman cussing because she had to spit her Skoal out.

"Where'd you say we was goin?" she asked as I led her down the hallway.

"To a program where they can help you get rid of those demons that are bothering you."

She smiled, a toothless one at that. "Any men up there?"

"Oh yeah," I laughed. "Yes ma'am, Ms. WiLou, you might just meet your match on this floor."

We entered the locked gates of Passages, the bright red ELOPEMENT sign still clinging to the entrance. As we passed the combination café / day room, I saw John sitting at one of the tables by himself, oblivious to the board games that the other patients were attempting to play under staff supervision. After conning WyLou to sit down across from the nursing station, I grabbed John's chart, hoping to find Baxter's psychiatric evaluation. As expected it hadn't been dictated and his hand-written note was not legible, providing no real clues at this point. His medication record also revealed nothing.

I turned and asked staff passing by about John and was rudely informed that his nurse was tied up with a patient. I almost got into an argument with the unit clerk but decided against it, realizing that if I angered too many staff, they'd run me off. With no clinical reason to be snooping around John's case, I eased back down the hall towards his table.

"John," I spoke softly, "you remember me?"

"From yesterday. You talked to me and Maggie didn't you?" He sat up, his eyes filled with anticipation. "Have you talked to her today? I miss her and need to be home. She's all alone."

I sat down next to him, avoiding eye contact with the unit staff. "I spoke with her this morning. She sends her love."

"Is she okay?" he asked with the bare bones honesty of a little boy worried about his best friend.

"She's fine," I said. "She told me to tell you how much she missed you and wants you home as soon as you get to feeling better."

"Michael, wasn't it?"

"Yes."

"Michael, other than feeling tired, thanks to my roommate, I'm fine. He's a real mess."

I scooted my chair closer to him. "What happened?"

"He tried to crawl into bed with me," John whispered, his eyes wide open.

"I'm sorry. Maybe I can suggest to the nurses to get you another room."

"Dr. Baxter said he would do that for me."

"You saw Dr. Baxter this morning?" I asked, edging even closer as the nursing staff eyeballed me from across the room.

"Yeah, I saw him. Still don't like him either."

"What'd he tell you about getting out?"

"That I needed to get well first and thought I could do that in a few days."

"Did he say anything else?"

"Yeah, about some disease or something. Said my bad dreams and forgetfulness were not just old age; that I might have something else, and he wanted to run some tests."

"Did he say what tests?"

"No, and I don't feel like staying here for another two or three days. I want to go home!"

"Shh..." I leaned in. "Let me see what I can find out."

"Can he keep me here against my will?"

"Unfortunately he can, at least for a few days. I'll check into it and get back to you later tonight. In the mean time, I'll call Maggie and let her know you're hanging in there."

"Please tell her I'm fine. I don't want her worrying. Besides..." He hung his head. "I feel bad about what I said to her last night."

"Last night?"

"When I kept telling her to get me out of here. I know she would have taken me home. I don't want her feeling bad. It's not her fault I'm in here."

"I'll tell her. Don't you worry, okay?"

"How'd she get home last night?" he asked. "I was scared to death about her driving by herself."

"She made it okay," I replied, reluctant to tell him that I'd followed her.

"But how'd she...?"

"She's a tough cookie," I said. "A lot like you." I patted him on his shoulder. "You hang in there okay? I'll see you later today." I started down the hallway.

"Will you call Maggie for me?" he called out.

"I'll call, I promise." I gave him the thumbs up sign and headed out the door.

chapter ten

I HUSTLED BACK TO THE OFFICE and was relieved to find that
the ER had no pending psych patients who needed to be
assessed. It was only ten in the morning, but I was drained as
I hobbled down the home stretch of my back-to-back-to-back
12-hour shifts, longing for my four days of seclusion from the
world, insane or otherwise. I'd grown accustomed to staying at
home, locked away with a handful of movies and a bucket of the
Colonel's finest, sometimes not even bothering to turn down the
bed sheets. On this day, however, as I basked in the momentary
reprieve from patients, I dreaded the thought of being at home
alone. For the first time in a long, long time, I was yearning for
human contact, if only for a day.

I heard the fumbling of keys on the other side of our office
door and reached behind me to open it, my moment of silence
ended.

"So you got her upstairs in one piece," Carol said, blowing
by me to the co-captain's chair, complete with papers scattered
in every direction and scratch sheets covered with artful doodles.

"She almost choked on her Skoal when I told her she couldn't
dip."

Carol refilled her coffee mug. "Did you see John while you were up there?"

I turned towards her. "It was sad."

"What happened?"

"He remembered me from last night," I said, sipping my store-bought sweet tea, "but as I was leaving, he lost it."

"How so?"

"He started repeating himself, as if our conversation only minutes earlier had never happened." I took a deep breath, slowly letting the air out. "I don't know…"

"Don't know what?" she asked as she logged back into her computer.

"I've seen it many times, but haven't felt it," I said as I fumbled with a twenty-one-page fax on a referral from an area hospital's ICU. "I mean I've felt it," I recanted. "I do have feelings, believe it or not."

Carol pulled back from her keyboard and faced me. "Makes sense."

"Meaning?" I held her gaze momentarily and then looked down, uncomfortable with the subject matter, especially around someone I was growing fonder of each day.

"You care about John and…"

"Maggie."

"They touched you deeply," she said, "for whatever reason."

I surveyed the empty assessment hallway with its dingy walls, dumpy furniture, and double-bagged paper bags overflowing with trash. I called our receptionist to cover us and motioned for Carol to follow me outside for a breath of fresh air. "We're eloping!" I announced to the psychiatric gods as I keyed the side entrance door and led her outside. "Think we got time to walk down to the pond?" I asked, overjoyed to feel the sunshine on my weary bones.

"Surely they can manage without us for fifteen minutes," she said.

We hustled to the far end of the lower parking lot and over a grassy knoll to a small but picturesque pond with a walking track around it.

"Is this where you run and hide?" Carol asked as we strolled alone on the hospital's best-kept secret. Since the pond-side entrance to the hospital was closed off several years ago, few people ventured down to the secluded area.

"As often as I can," I replied, "which hasn't been much of late."

"So now I know where to find you," she said, playfully bumping into me.

"Didn't know you were looking."

"You never know..." Carol looked up, her eyes sparkling against the backdrop of a cloudless Carolina-blue sky. "So tell me about this old couple that has touched your life," she said. "What makes them so special?"

"Fifty-six years of marriage, for one," I said as I wandered down to the edge of the pond. "I should have brought some bread."

"Bread?" she asked.

"You've never seen the turtles in here?" I playfully scolded.

"I don't see any turtles."

"Bring some bread next time, and I'll show you turtles."

We stepped away from the water's edge and watched as a Mama duck led her three offspring across the pond.

Carol turned to face me. "So what is it about John and Maggie?"

"What," I stepped back, "you turned investigative reporter on me?"

"No, but they've opened up a side of you that I sensed was always there."

"Oh yeah?" I folded my arms across my chest. "What side is that?"

"A compassionate, caring side as opposed to the hardened old man."

"Hardened I might agree with," I said, "but did you have to throw in the old man part?"

"If the shoe fits…" She grinned.

"Some friend you are." I turned back towards the track.

"Hey!" Carol grabbed my arm, spinning me around, "You're the best looking old coot I've seen in a long time." She stood there gazing at me.

For a brief moment I thought about kissing her but chickened out, not knowing what to do. I started walking, haphazardly throwing my arm around her. "Guess I should take that as a compliment, huh?"

"Better take what you can get at our age," she said. "Now, are you going to tell me about them, or am I left to wonder?"

I plopped down on the park bench. "Yesterday was the first time I've allowed myself to get personally involved," I said, looking out at the pond, "and it felt good."

"Excuse me," Carol said, "did you say feel?"

"I said felt, smart-ass."

"Short-lived, I assume," she fired back. "Go on."

I was momentarily speechless, the art of verbal jabbing in the office one thing, but outside the office and with a potential partner. I felt like I was back in junior high, fearful of making a fool of myself.

She sat down next to me. "Come on." She touched my forearm. "I want to hear what happened."

"How many hundreds of cases over the past two years?" I wondered aloud as I took a deep breath and turned to face her. "I said all the right things in my yeoman's best Hollywood performance. Yesterday," I propped my left knee on the bench,

"I let my guard down when Maggie told me their story. I don't know why. Yeah, well, I do know why."

Carol smiled, encouraging me to continue.

"They remind me so much of my parents." I blurted out. "And Maggie is my Mom made over. I only wish…"

Carol reached over and touched my hand.

"They're a dying breed," I said, unable to hold her gaze, "especially Maggie." I stopped, wondering how she'd react if I told her what I'd done. I decided to take a chance.

"You what?" She pulled her hand back.

"I followed Maggie home last night."

"Why?"

"She was scared to death!" I countered. "Beyond the fact that she rarely drives, imagine spending every waking moment with someone you love for fifty-six years."

"Seventeen years 'bout killed me," she said, "not to mention what I wanted to do to my ex."

"He's not buried in your backyard is he?"

"Way too close for comfort," she grinned. "So, you followed her home. Then what? Did she show you his briefs or…?"

"His balls," I deadpanned. "One ball actually. That's all he ever wanted."

"I should have figured," she fired back. "That wild woman you saw this morning got you all hot and bothered." What was her name?"

"WyLoooo," I howled. "It was the Skoal juice oozing down her hairy chin that excited me."

"You are sick aren't you?" she teased.

"Especially when I'm holdin' one ball," I said in my finest Southern drawl.

"You obviously are dying to tell me about his ball, or balls."

"Ever hear of Joltin' Joe?" I asked.

"Ever hear of the Yankee Clipper?" she shot back, stealing my home-run pitch.

"You know DiMaggio?" I gestured.

"I know DiMaggio," she said, her face aglow in the sunlight.

"John's got a baseball signed by none other," I said. "One of my father's heroes."

"My Dad too," Carol said, a peaceful look in her eyes. "He'd tell me stories about DiMaggio and how he was the game's most complete player."

We sat in silence as a slate-blue heron glided across the pond and eased to a stop, his spindly legs hunkered down in the shallows near a family of mallards snoozing underneath the shade of a weeping willow, whose branches tickled the water.

"So what's next for John and Maggie?" she asked, breaking our silence.

I glanced at my watch and stood. "I don't know. I just hate to see Baxter sink his grubby research claws into them."

We started back towards the hospital.

"Back to insanity," she said, nudging me.

I draped my arm around her. "That's what we live for ain't it?"

She stopped as we approached the clearing and turned towards me. "Can we do this again some time?"

I smiled. "I'd like that very much."

"Me too."

Back in the office, I took a moment to call Maggie. I didn't have the heart to tell her about John's memory lapse and wasn't about to drop Baxter's bomb of some degenerative disease of the brain. I figured he was making reference to Alzheimer's, but I didn't feel like scaring her at this point. She needed to hear something positive, so I opted to share his message of love and concern for her. I also assured her that I would check on him later and call her with an update.

The remainder of our afternoon was a blur as the non-stop parade of frequent-flyers waltzed in for their usual end-of-the-month tune-ups. As sundown approached, Faith General swayed to the sounds of a hostile psychotic beat. Every unit in the hospital, both medical and psychiatric, was at or near capacity, stretching front-line staff beyond their limits, igniting the simmering coals of hostility among patients on the adult acute psych unit.

"Code 100, plaza five," the hospital operator coldly announced overhead. "Code 100, plaza five."

I was in the ER interviewing an ornery alcoholic when the door to the interview room flew open. It was Ralph, the evening maintenance man and first backup to our security staff — a staff of one. "Don't mean to interrupt, but can you go with me up to plaza five? Security's up checking the boiler, and we ain't got but a handful of guys working tonight."

I let my patient meander back out to the lobby and jogged along behind Ralph, all the while praying that I would not be needed in the fray. We hopped off the elevator, unlocked the door to plaza five and hustled down the hallway, Ralph five yards ahead of me. I rounded the corner to find several of the nurses locked in the nursing station.

"What's going on?" I questioned, out of breath from my brief scamper.

"We're okay," the nurse replied. "James from geri-psych and four other staff from downstairs are holding her down in seclusion. We're waiting on the doctor to call us back so we can give her a shot."

"Shoot who?" Ralph snapped.

"She came in last night strung out on crystal meth."

"Crystal what?" Ralph asked as he started out the door towards the seclusion room.

"Hard to say if it's drug induced," the nurse said. "Either

way, she's hallucinating, and huge. Weighs about two fifty and not afraid to throw a punch."

"What set her off?" I asked, feeling obligated to follow Ralph out to where the action was, hoping, as the nurses handed me latex gloves, that the action was long over and I could return to my mealy-mouthed drunk in the ER.

"She's used to bullying to get her way," the nurse replied, "and a little on the schizoid side. If that's not enough, I got seven other acutely psychotic patients up here and no male tech."

"Makes us the crazy ones for working here," a female tech sneered.

My prayer was answered as I turned the hallway corner and found five brave staff holding the wild-eyed woman down. Ralph jumped in for good measure. Chemical reinforcement came only minutes later as a nurse popped the acutely psychotic patient with a geodon/ativan cocktail.

I strolled back to the nursing station, tossed my latex gloves into the garbage can like a hot-shot doctor coming out of surgery, wiped my brow, and headed out the door.

"Thanks for your help," Terri called out, unaware that I'd done nothing more than watch the real warriors at work.

"No problem." I was once again relieved that I'd weaseled out of restraining a patient. I'd done my time grappling with aggressive clients. Twelve years in a state hospital with emotionally disturbed teens had taken its toll.

Since the ER had no one waiting to be assessed and my patient was not suicidal and had probably gone out to his truck to smoke a cigarette and down another shot of booze, I felt no great rush to get back to him. Instead, I stopped in to check on John. I was greeted by the church lady, beseeching me to let her out before the demons destroyed her. I redirected her back towards the far end of the unit and entered the group room where most of the others were finishing supper. Three patients clutched the chair railing as they shuffled about the hallway. James, their nurse for the shift, had gone up to plaza five to assist in the code 100. As soon as he left, staff had to break up a cat fight between two female patients, both in their seventies. The unit was in bedlam as the lone remaining tech hustled to feed those requiring assistance and clean up a variety of messes before the evening shift arrived.

I spotted John in the back, sitting alone at the same table where I'd talked to him earlier.

"Hey John!" I patted him on the shoulder. How are you feeling?"

"Not good."

"You remember me don't you?" I asked with a smile, hoping not to offend him.

"Yeah, I remember," he snapped. "Why do you keep asking?"

"I'm just concerned about you." I sat down across from him.

"If you're so concerned," John said, "then why can't you get me out of here?"

"That's up to Dr. Baxter," I said. "Has he come by again?"

"About an hour ago, I think it was. What time is it anyway?"

I glanced at my watch. "Almost six o'clock," I said. "What'd he say?"

"Who?" he snarled, pushing his half-eaten tray away in disgust. I could relate, having devoured Maggie's cooking late last night.

"Dr. Baxter?" I asked.

"He told me I couldn't leave, that he could keep me here against my will for a week and there was nothing I could do about it. Is that true?"

"Unfortunately, yes," I said, turning my chair away from the nursing station. "He can hold you up to ninety-six hours, or four days."

John shook his head in disgust. "What happens then?"

"If the patient hasn't signed a voluntary consent for treatment by then, the case goes before a judge downtown."

"Then what?"

"As I understand it, you have the right to an attorney, or the courts appoint one for you. The hospital attorneys and physician are also there, and each side presents its case. The judge then decides if the patient can be held an additional fifteen days against his will, or he may rule that the patient no longer meets emergency commitment criteria and must be set free immediately."

"Sounds like the patient doesn't have a chance," he said, a dejected look on his face.

"I've never been to one of those hearings, so I really don't know what happens," I said. "But, yeah, you got docs and hospital attorneys on one side and a patient on the other. The odds are stacked against the patient in most cases."

"That's the feeling I got too," John replied, appearing as lucid as I'd seen him since we met.

"The other alternative," I said, "is to consent to treatment and participate in the program. Then, in most cases, you're out in a week, sometimes less. If you're not exhibiting any behaviors that are considered dangerous to yourselves or others, the hospital is hard-pressed to hold you against your will beyond seventy-two hours."

"You sound like Baxter," he snapped.

"I'm not trying to persuade you one way or the other," I said. "I just know you're caught in the middle here. You're too high functioning to be on this unit and don't belong on any of the other units around here. Yet, no one, including myself, wants to send you home without some sense of safety…" I hesitated for a moment, but knew I had to finish. "That's the bottom line John, some level of reassurance that you won't go after Maggie again with a knife. We want ya'll to be safe."

He had a pained look on his face, as if reliving the events of yesterday afternoon for the first time. He sat motionless, and I wondered if he was losing touch with reality again. He looked up at me, sadness in his eyes. "I wouldn't hurt Maggie. I love her and miss her so much." He stopped to clear his throat and regain his composure. "I believe what you and Maggie have told me — that I thought she was an intruder and I went after her with a butcher knife. I know you're not lying to me. But..." He hesitated again, tears welling up in his eyes. "I can't remember what happened. I just don't know..." He hung his head as the chaos played out all around us, staff and the other patients oblivious to our table.

I wasn't sure what to do except reach up and put my hand on his shoulder. I couldn't imagine the pain and anguish he felt, knowing deep in his heart that his mind was playing the worst kind of tricks on him.

"John, I wish I had a simple answer, but I don't. I do know that Maggie can't wait to have you back home where you belong. In the mean time, think about signing a voluntary consent for treatment. Do the time, so to speak, and get the heck out in one piece."

He looked up and smiled, his eyes meeting mine, his gaze telling me that he appreciated my straightforward honesty with him. "What do you think about his research project?" he asked.

"I don't know much about it," I said. "Baxter is supposedly known nationally for his work with the elderly, but I don't know the details of what he's doing."

"He wants me to become a part of his Alzheimer's study."

I was surprised by his matter-of-fact comment. If Baxter asked him to take part in his research, then the good doctor felt that John's symptoms were severe enough to diagnose him with the dreaded disease. That, or he needed subjects and was recruiting any and all takers. I wouldn't put that past him, even though I had no reason to believe Baxter was unethical.

"So what'd you tell him?" I asked.

"Told him sure, why not. If it gets me out faster, I'll do it."

"What do you have to do?"

"He's starting me on an experimental treatment in the next day or two," John said. "He wants me to agree to stay on the drug for ten weeks."

"Ten weeks?"

"Yeah, I'd continue taking it at home and agree to come in for re-checks in his office every two weeks."

"So you already told him you'd do it?" I asked, observing as James returned from Plaza five and immediately started redirecting wandering patients in the hallway.

"Signed the papers just a little while ago," he replied.

"So why were you asking me about the committal stuff?"

He leaned in. "I wanted to know the truth," he whispered. "I don't trust Baxter. I do trust you."

"Why me?" I asked.

"Cause Maggie told me what you did last night, that's why."

I looked at him with surprise, his candor catching me off guard.

He sat straight up. "You didn't have to do what you did, and I appreciate that," he said. "Maggie did too."

I nodded my head, my insides dancing with delight.

John continued. "You rarely come across people anymore willing to go out of their way. She was scared to death about the drive home, and you took care of that even though you'd already worked a 13-hour day." He calmly pointed at me. "And you didn't even know us. That, my friend, is a class human being."

I leaned back in my chair and smiled. It was the first genuine compliment about me as a human being that I'd heard in a long time. I wasn't about to dismiss my feelings of joy too soon.

"I have to ask," John said. "You didn't get any smudges on my baseball did ya?"

"No sir," I smiled. "That's quite a catch — a baseball signed by Joe DiMaggio. You ever see him play?"

He leaned back in his chair and, for one shining moment, forgot where he was. "No, son, I sure didn't, but what a joy it was to watch the newsreels and listen on the radio. He glided around centerfield. Everything was effortless for him. He'd make the toughest catch or stretch a single into a double with such ease you'd wonder why the other players wouldn't do the same. It was only after you followed him enough to know that the other players didn't do it because they couldn't do what Joe did. He just did it with such grace. There may have been better players but I sure didn't see them."

"Not even Ted Williams?" I challenged him.

"A better hitter, yes, Williams was the greatest hitter I ever saw, bar none. But better all-around player? No, Williams couldn't do all the things that DiMaggio did to win a ballgame. Nobody did."

"He was before my time," I said. "My dad loved him and said the same thing — that DiMaggio was poetry in motion in every phase of the game. But the greatest?" I hesitated. "I would have to go with Willie Mays, the 'say hey' kid. He could do it all with such flare."

"That's a toss-up," John replied. "Mays was a great hitter and covered a lot of ground in centerfield."

"He could run too," I said. "Stole a lot of bases over his career."

"Yeah, but I'd still take Joe as my starting centerfielder."

"You sound like my old man," I said with a smile, reliving those wonderful childhood moments when my father and I watched ballgames together.

"So your father was a DiMaggio fan?" John asked.

"Oh yeah, a big time fan," I said, "although, we used to argue over Mays and Mantle. I loved Mays, and Pop loved Mantle. He always said if Mickey hadn't been hurt he would have broken all the records."

"Ol' Mick might have done it, that's true. He was a heckuva ballplayer."

As the staff flitted around cleaning up the aftermath and shuffling patients to their rooms, John and I sat back and savored the moment, both of us reliving a piece of the past as only America's pastime can offer — a glimpse back to a simpler time, a time with genuine heroes, and a brief moment away from the harsh realities of locked units and degenerative brain diseases.

"We let people live too long anymore," John said. "I don't want to live just to exist somewhere," he continued. "I guess that's every old person's wish — to live a full life and die in their sleep before all the diseases and disgraces of old age set in."

I didn't have an answer for him and didn't feel like I needed one. Like two old friends sitting on a park bench, we sat in silence as WiLou and the 92-year-old Viagra man teetered towards her room while the church lady roamed the hall, imploring all to come to the Father.

An hour later, I was done with my work-week and ready to roll. Yearning to talk to Carol, I hung around the office for a few minutes, only to succumb to my comfort zone and drinking at home alone. I wasn't ready to share my KFC and Jack Daniels, much less my TV buttons.

chapter eleven

"WELCOME BACK STRANGER," CAROL SAID with a smile. "We missed you around here."

"Wish I could say the same," I replied as I dropped my old backpack and plopped down in the captain's cubicle next to her. "Actually, I did miss this place, parts of it." I smiled back at her. She looked good, even better than before for some reason. Maybe my senses were coming alive again, I don't know, but, man, she looked real good at the moment. I wondered if she knew what I was thinking.

"You ain't right if you missed this place," said David, scrambling to secure his paperwork and escort his patient upstairs. "I've seen several of your favorites in the past two days alone."

"Bipolar and borderline, of course."

"Every last one of 'em!" David cackled, poking Carol in the ribs. "Where would I be without my borderline buddies?"

"Probably going out with them," Carol jabbed back.

"At least going somewhere," I mumbled.

Carol turned her attention back my way. "So you holed up in your apartment for four days and what — watched a dozen movies?"

"Six," I sneered.

Carol shook her head. "You're pitiful, you know."

"Sounds like an anti-social personality disorder to me," David teased as he grabbed the phone to notify the stress unit of their new admission.

She handed me a cup of coffee. "You stayed in the entire time you were off?"

"I had to go out and get the movies!" I fired back, elated that she seemed interested enough to care. "Seriously, I did get out and walk two days. And..."

"And?" She playfully tilted her head.

"I bought a bike!" I said, beaming like the joy-filled carefree kid I used to be.

Carol's face lit up. "You're kidding?"

"A good ol' street bike," I said. "The kind you pedal."

"I know what you're referring to," she said with a grin. "I love to ride. Or..."

"Or what?" I playfully snapped. Yeah, I knew she loved to ride, but I bought it for me. Sort of. At the time, however, I was imagining the two of us riding off into a brilliant sunset, Carol on her fifteen-hundred-dollar touring bike and me on my two hundred dollar Sears special.

"So when are you going to ride with me?" Carol popped the question.

"Thought you'd never ask," I sarcastically replied.

"You big chicken!" She whacked me on my arm. "Too afraid to ask me out so you get me to do it for you. What kind of man are you?"

"Probably bipolar, with a tinge of borderline," I teased, "but I ain't no..."

David cackled from the back copy machine as Jo, our supervisor, walked in.

"You guys!" Jo laughed. "You know the rumors are flying about this department again don't you?"

"Rumors?" David asked, always eager to hear the latest gossip. "What are we doing now?"

"Sneaking off and taking romantic walks around the pond," Jo said with a smile. "I can't imagine anyone on our assessment team doing such a thing, can you?"

"If that's all they got," I said, "then we're in pretty good shape."

"Especially now," Jo said.

"Did I miss something while I was off?" I asked.

"No one's filled you guys in yet?" she asked, turning to my comrades.

"We're the last to know anything outside of the ER," said Carol. "What happened?"

"We had a patient die up on the geri-psych unit around midnight last night, a male."

"What?" I stammered, my heart suddenly racing, head pounding, mouth dry as a bone.

"You alright?" Carol asked.

I nodded and turned back to Jo. "What was his name?"

"I don't know," Jo replied. "He was part of that Alzheimer's research project."

"What happened?" I asked, turning back to Carol. "Will you pull the geri-psych census up please?"

"I heard the guy died from a heart attack," Jo said. "Makes you wonder."

"And?" I demanded, glaring at Carol's computer screen, praying John's name popped up.

Jo, kind soul that she was, didn't take my abruptness personally. "The question on everyone's mind — was he on the new experimental drug, the vaccine for Alzheimer's?"

"C'mon computer!" I cried.

"Is Baxter up there killing patients off?" asked David.

"I don't believe this," Carol moaned as her screen went blank. "Michael…"

I bolted out the door and down the ER hallway, bypassing the elevators for the stairs. Two at a time, I scampered up four flights, panting as I reached the entrance to the second floor hallway. My heart pumping, my thoughts racing, I stood in the eerie silence of the stairwell, trying to catch my breath and my composure.

Surely my friend was okay. I couldn't recall Maggie mentioning heart problems. She'd said something about a blood pressure medication, but that's not unusual for a man in his seventies. And surely Baxter had ruled out any patients with potential reactions to side effects. Wouldn't he have to? Yet, someone has already died! Is it coincidence, or did the patient have a reaction to some experimental medication?

I grabbed the door handle, took two deep breaths and entered the hallway leading to the geriatric psychiatric unit. With a death on the unit, not to mention the chaos of the code blue medical team rushing onto the floor in an attempt to revive the man, the patients, at least the ones with some sense of reality left, had to be spooked.

I stopped at the locked doors leading in, wondering if I was prepared to find out if John was the one. How would I tell Maggie? What would I tell her? She trusted me to look out for him. I swiped my badge and opened the door.

"Repent and be healed evil one!" cried the church lady as she grabbed my hand and coerced me down the hall towards her room.

I played along, taking every opportunity to look for John as we paraded past the day room towards the nursing station. Onward we marched in slow motion as I peeked into every room along the way. Still no sign of him.

"Where's John?" I asked the church lady in desperation.

"John the Baptist?"

"No, John the patient."

"Married to Maggie?" she replied, a gleam in her haunting brown eyes.

"Yes!" I squeezed her hand and stopped, startled that she would know about Maggie unless...

"Oh, he's gone."

"Gone?"

"Gone to see God," she wistfully laughed, pulling on me to continue down the hall.

"Where?" I stopped, freeing my hand from her grasp.

"To the pond to see God!" She pointed out the door, laughed again, and cut loose with a strange, eerie shriek. "Repent ye vile serpents! The time is near. Repent!" She pointed her long, bony finger at me, smiled and waltzed away.

"What's up?" asked Sally, my favorite nurse on the unit.

"Been off a few days and thought I'd check on a patient I admitted last week."

"What's his name?"

"John Dalton."

"He's not here," she said, checking their patient board. "Wait a minute. He's the one..."

"What?" I blurted out. "I'm sorry." I forced a smile.

"Rough morning down in the pit, huh?"

"Just tell me. Is John alive?"

"What?" Sally cried. "You know something I don't because he was standing right here in front of me fifteen minutes ago."

I stood speechless, a strange sensation warming me, flashes of my father, who passed away fifteen years ago, smiling at me.

"You okay, Michael?" Sally asked.

"Yeah," I graciously nodded. "I just didn't know..."

She studied my face, ever the intuitive compassionate nurse. "You heard about the death and thought it was your friend."

"Patient," I corrected her.

"Yeah, well to hear John and his wife talk, I'd say you're more like family to them," Sally replied. "They think the world of you. You okay? You still aren't looking like yourself."

"Yeah, I'm fine," I said. "Sorry I jumped."

"No need," she smiled. "Now, let me see…" She checked the log. "Looks like he's gone for a walk around the pond. Jimmy took them out about ten minutes ago."

"I'll be." I laughed aloud as I glanced down the hallway where the church lady was working her magic on her congregation, in this case, an old man facing the wall, rocking repetitively back and forth. "She's something," I muttered.

"What?" Sally asked.

"Oh, nothing. Thanks Sally."

I stopped by the assessment office to make sure all was well and headed across the parking lot. From a distance I could see the crew creeping along on the far side of the walking track. I finally caught up to them as they stopped to feed the turtles.

"Where have you been?" he asked with a big smile, extending his hand.

"It's my first day back," I said, clasping his firm handshake. "Went upstairs to find you."

"Thought I'd escaped, huh?"

We walked away from the pond towards a bench just a few feet away from the trail.

"Worse than that," I replied. "What I meant…"

"I know what you meant," he said, sitting down on the bench. "It scared me too."

I nodded, surprised by his candor. We watched as the others tossed bread crumbs to the turtles gathered near the edge of the pond. "So how are you feeling?" I asked.

"Much better."

"That's good to here."

"Must have been my blood pressure," he said with a sly smile.

"You think so?" I asked, wondering what he was thinking, or perhaps hiding.

"I'm fine. How 'bout you?" he asked. "That's a nice schedule you got — a three-day work week."

"I like it. Those twelve to thirteen hour days are rough, but it's great having four days off," I said, still curious but cautious, not wanting to upset him out here. After three years of fighting with hospital administration and the doctors, patients had finally earned the right, with a doctor's order of course, to leave their respective locked units and take supervised walks outside. I wasn't about to take a chance on that privilege getting pulled again. "So how's Maggie?" I asked.

"She's doing great! Our daughter came to town to stay with her while I'm stuck down here. They came to see me over the weekend."

"Where's your daughter live?"

"In Hendersonville, North Carolina, near Asheville. We can't get her to leave those mountains. She stayed after her divorce, not wanting to move the kids away from their friends. I don't understand it."

"What's that?" I asked, reaching down for a clover.

"Why your generation can't keep a marriage together," he replied. "You're divorced aren't you?"

"How'd you know?"

"Maggie told me. Said you have a son."

"Just turned twenty-one."

"You close to him?" John asked.

"No, can't say that I am," I said, studying the miniscule three-leaf clover.

"Why not?" He fired back.

I was tempted to throw his son up in his face but resisted

and gave him a condensed version of my screwed-up life and marriage.

"Yeah, greed and the almighty dollar can take a man down," he replied. "That's what happened to my daughter. Her husband fell in love with the road and the riches along the way and forgot about his family."

"So when are you busting out of this joint?" I asked.

"Dr. Qualls seems to think I'm okay to leave tomorrow."

"Dr. Qualls?" I said, surprised. "How'd you wind up with him?"

"What? You don't like him?" he asked with a mischievous grin.

I looked at him and laughed, sensing that he knew what I was thinking. "No, I like him just fine, what dealings I've had with him anyway. He just..." I stopped. "What happened to Baxter?"

"Guess he was too busy, so he sent his cohort in to tend to us guinea pigs." John couldn't hold back his emotions as he let out a hearty laugh, startling the others who approached.

"Guinea pigs?" I said as the tech motioned that it was time to go.

"Okay if Michael walks me up in a few minutes?" John asked.

"That's fine with me. You okay with that, Michael?"

"No problem."

"Hope I'm not imposing," John said, leaning back on the bench.

"Not at all," I replied. "So you haven't seen Baxter?"

"Not since he threatened to commit me if I didn't sign in."

"Is he seeing any of the patients up there?"

"I haven't seen him."

"So do you like Dr. Qualls?"

"He's alright, I guess. Spends five minutes a day with me. Asks me how I'm feeling, stuff like that, and then he's on his merry way. He's an odd man, no doubt about it."

"How so?" I asked, curious about his perception of the doctor we in the assessment office referred to as Dr. Quack. He waddled down the hospital hallways like a duck and seemed to be out in left field about half of the time, often forgetting that he'd already been paged and had taken report on patients from the assessment office. He was popular among the bipolar bunch, always willing to prescribe xanax, a highly addictive benzodiazepine, for anxiety. It wasn't uncommon for some of his long-standing patients to wind up on our addictions unit.

John grinned. "I don't know. He just goes off on a tangent right in the middle of a conversation."

"That he does," I said, thinking how ironic that a man supposedly with Alzheimer's and on a locked geriatric psychiatric unit had the wherewithal to know that his psychiatrist is a fruitcake. I chose not to pursue the subject further, but my guess was that Baxter needed a doctor he could easily manipulate and control to do the day-to-day stuff — making rounds, writing the notes, and so forth. He had his research coordinator there to keep an eye on Qualls. That way, Baxter was free to pursue other research possibilities and remain one step removed from the experiment, even though his research protocols were probably laid out so that Qualls could do very little to screw things up. Or so it seemed.

"So you're leaving in the next few days, huh?" I asked.

"Can't wait," John replied as he stood up. "Guess we better get back. I don't want to upset the fruit cart up there, you know?"

We meandered around the track towards the parking lot, John delighted that he would be back home soon with Maggie and her home cooking.

"She's a pretty good cook huh," he said with a grin.

"Best meal I've had in a long time."

He stopped and gently grabbed my arm. "I'll always be grateful for what you did the other night."

I patted him on the back. "My privilege."

"You'll have to come out for supper one night soon," he said. "I'd like for you to see Maggie again and meet my daughter."

"I'd be honored."

We strolled along like two old friends, stopping along the creek-like drainage area filled with tadpoles and frogs. To our right and up the hill a family of squirrels scampered about the pines while a solitary red-tailed hawk circled ominously above.

"Yes sir, I can't wait to get back home." John gazed up the hill at the serene surroundings. "I miss my backyard and Maggie's beautiful flowers." He smiled. "Sure miss her coffee too 'bout this time every morning."

"I'm going to miss you," I said, "but I'm sure glad you're getting out."

"You mean alive don't you?" he quipped.

His comment surprised me. I'd wanted to ask him about the death on the unit, but was reluctant to do so. Turns out I didn't need to.

"That man who died last night," John said, "I heard the nurses say that he didn't have any family left to take care of him. Apparently he mistreated his wife and kids for years, and they finally disowned him. Guess they'd had enough. Sad to think of spending your last breath with no family around."

"What happened to him?" I asked, his comment hitting home.

"I heard he had a heart attack."

"Was he part of the research group?" I asked.

"I think he was," he replied. "That's been kind of hush-hush. I'd heard that there were eight of us guinea pigs, but I don't really know for sure who the others are. I know everyone on the unit was spooked when it happened. Even some of the staff."

"Like who?"

"Ms. Farmer, the nurse in charge, was real upset and shaky."

"Do they have you on medication?" I asked.

He nodded.

"What is it?"

"Don't know," he abruptly said, turning his attention back towards the trees.

I waited to see if he'd say anymore but he didn't. Rarely, if ever for that matter, had a geri-psych patient been admitted and not placed on some type of medication. Most were on a garden variety of pharmaceutical concoctions geared to combat their medical problems, memory loss, delusions or sudden violent outbursts. I looked up at John, wondering if he was on some experimental Alzheimer's vaccine, or perhaps nothing more than his hypertension meds and a sugar pill placebo.

We made it to the entrance of the hospital, both of us reluctant to let go of the fresh air and sunshine. As we approached the geri-psych unit, he stopped and turned to me. "I can't thank you enough."

"My pleasure," I said, shaking his hand. "I'll see you again soon."

"Maggie and I are counting on that."

I escorted him down to the nursing station, the hallway unusually quiet.

"I see you found your friend," Sally said. "Did you have a good walk?"

"Glorious." John winked at me. "When can I go again?"

"We'll see if we can sneak you back out later today," she replied.

"Can't wait," John said and meandered towards his favorite table in the day room.

I headed back to the pit, hoping all was quiet on our psychiatric home front, wondering if Baxter had something to hide.

Like a dead body.

chapter twelve

"YES!" I WHISPERED WITH JOY as I scanned the empty ER waiting room. "My favorite scene," I said in passing to the evening admissions registrar hunkered down in her barren cubicle.

"What's with the Bubba grin?" Carol teased from the ER nursing station where first shift RN's rollicked with Dr. Mac, their favorite ER doc, all enjoying the brief reprieve from patients.

"Did Watson get laid last night?" Dr. Mac's voice bellowed down the hallway.

"I wish…" I muttered, glad to see Carol headed my way.

"You getting out on time tonight?" she asked in passing.

"Looks good at the moment," I said. "Why?"

"Just wondering." She shot me a smile. "I was hoping to leave early if it's not too crazy."

"What's the occasion?"

"Dinner at El Chico's," she said. "I've got a gift certificate that's about to expire. You like Mexican?"

I smiled. "Does a bear…?"

"What?"

"An old saying," I said. "Guess you're not old enough."

"Or redneck enough," she fired back. "Hurry up so we can get out before the floodgates open."

"I'm all for that."

What have I gotten myself into? I pondered as I pulled out of the hospital parking lot, Carol's car leading the way to my first non-work-related encounter with a respectable woman since my wife left me four years earlier. I sneered, flashbacks of many an anguished night all alone, my insides boiling with betrayal.

I changed the radio station to smooth jazz, hoping to chill my labile nerves as I pulled into the restaurant parking lot. I circled the lot, grateful that there were no parking spaces next to Carol. I parked and checked my ever-graying hair in the rearview mirror one last time before easing out of my car.

Carol walked over to me. "Ever been here before?"

"No." I stepped back, tongue-tied for the moment, mesmerized at the sight of her in a sleek, Indian-styled blouse with her hair hanging free and her cowboy boots a testament to her free-spirit.

I almost sat down on the same side of the booth but caught myself and slid in across from her. What few encounters I had mustered with the female gender over the past several years were not with women I'd sit on either side of the booth with, much less take home to meet Mom.

"You remember how to eat in public don't you?" Carol teased.

"It's been awhile."

"You poor neglected soul. You got some catching up to do."

"Yeah, well, on my salary," I said, glancing over the top of my menu at her, "it may take awhile."

She pulled back slowly, holding her gaze on me. "I thought you were some corporate hotshot before you came here."

"Another lifetime," I replied, momentarily lost in thought. "Made a decent living back then." I laid the menu down and reached for my drink. "Loved the people and the job. So much so that I lost my family."

She scooted the bowl of chips and dip closer to me. "How so?"

I shared my story with her and my four year fall from grace, blurring that mystical entity known as truth somewhere between fact and perception.

"A 21-year-old son, huh," she said.

I dipped my chip in the hot salsa and took a big bite. "Yep," I said, "hopefully wiser than his old man."

"Does he look like you?"

"Used to, or so I was told," I said. "I haven't seen him in two years."

"Why not?"

"You have kids don't you?" I asked, hoping to change the focus.

"Two girls, both away in college, but I still talk to them every week."

"So where's their father?" I cross-examined.

"In Atlanta, with his new wife and family," she smirked.

"I'm sorry," I said."

She sipped her Margarita. "He has little to do with them anymore, yet the girls think he hung the moon. I'm the one who busted it to keep a roof over their heads when dear old dad's business was faltering and he was too busy…" She hesitated, taking another long drink. "He's the hero and I'm just Mom. That's what my girls say to me. 'Oh Mother, you'll always be there.' But let Daddy invite them down for a weekend and he's the greatest thing since…"

I tipped my mug to her and took a long slow drink, prepared to plead the fifth if she aimed her angry rant my way.

"How come you good-for-nothing men get all the glory and we do all the work?"

"It's in our genes," I smirked. "That male lion mentality."

She dangled a chip over the cheese sauce. "More like

impotent male ego mentality." She dipped and chomped down on her chip. "I'm not letting you off that easy."

I ran my finger along the salt-rimmed edge of my glass, trying to recall the last time I drank Margaritas in a frozen beer mug. "Meaning?" I asked.

"So what's up with your son?" she quizzed. "You think he doesn't want to see his old man?"

"He's still angry about our divorce," I said, licking the salt off my finger. "He blames me for not being there, and frankly, I can't argue with him. I wasn't around much the last six or seven years."

"When he was, what, fifteen or sixteen," Carol said, "and really needed a father?"

"You don't have to rub my nose in it."

She leaned in. "What are you doing to rectify the situation?"

I shrugged my shoulders. "He's not ready. He made that all very clear the last time I saw him."

"What's he doing now?"

"He's still in school at U-T and working part-time," I said. "He's a good kid. He'll land on his feet."

"Like his old man."

"No," I said, "far better than his old man." I downed my Margarita and reached for the happy hour pitcher.

Carol held her mug out. "So what's so bad about your life?"

I filled her glass to the brim. "It's humbling to go back to the front lines, but I'm enjoying the challenge and loving the 12-hour shifts." I refilled my mug and set the empty pitcher down. "I just don't see myself working in a psychiatric ER for the next ten years."

"What do you wanna do?"

"I don't know," I said. "I'm just now picking myself up off the canvass." I tipped my mug. "Thanks partly to you."

"Me?" She was the one blushing this time.

"You have a purpose outside of the pit," I said. "A passion."

"I do?" She leaned forward, an intriguing look on her face.

"You've got your three-day work-week that pays the bills," I said, "giving you the other four days to pursue your art and painting. That's what you live for isn't it?"

She beamed. "How'd you know that?"

"I watch when you're on the phone or there's down time," I said. "If you're not drawing or doodling, you're reading about it."

She leaned across the table, playfully whispering, "You sure have a strange way of letting someone know you're interested."

"Yeah, well," I flagged the waiter down, "I've come to appreciate strange over the past few years." I handed the waiter the empty pitcher and chip bowl.

"Just as long as you're not peeping Tom strange."

"That's a thought," I said, a coy smile on my face.

"You're sick, old man," she replied with a devilish grin.

"What'd you expect?" I clutched my drink. "Look at who I spend all my time with."

She reached over and patted my hand. "We need to get you out more often."

I nodded and smiled. "Sounds good to me."

We ate and conversed, my insides tingling. I wondered if Carol was feeling the same, her sultry eyes growing more inviting with each savored bite.

"What time do you go in tomorrow?" she asked.

"The usual. Seven a.m. How 'bout you?"

"Tomorrow's my crazy shift."

"Ten to ten?"

"You got it," she replied.

"I'll save you a drunk or two."

"Better an addict than a whiny female that early in the morning," she said.

Must be nice to sleep in," I said.

"Oh, I'll be up."

"Yeah, right," I said. "Doing what?"

"Doodling as you call it," she said. "There's nothing like the early morning light, the birds singing, and…"

"And?"

"Just me and my painting," she said. "That's what I live for, remember?"

"Sounds peaceful."

She leaned back and smiled, her eyes revealing her joy. "The greatest feeling in the world. As if time didn't exist some days."

"Must be nice to have that artistic outlet," I said. "I can't draw or paint a thing."

"You'd be surprised what you could do with a little coaching."

I was dying to say, 'Great! Let's get started tonight!' but I didn't have the nerve to be so bold. Instead, we fumbled over the bill and walked out to the parking lot. Suddenly I was fourteen and at the Tennessee Theatre, clueless as to how to kiss the girl, my best buddy and his gal already lost in a French kissing marathon.

"Well, I guess this is it," I mumbled. "Thanks for the…"

Before I could finish, she pulled me in and kissed me on the lips, a brief but passionate one indeed. She stepped back, gazing at me standing there like a bumbling idiot.

"You okay?" She reached up to touch my cheek. "I hope I…"

I pulled her into a bear hug, electricity roaring through my veins.

"Hey," she whispered in my ear.

"Yeah." I held on tight.

"I can't breathe."

She exhaled as I let go, her hand still clutching mine. "You done this very often?"

"Every night before I go to bed," I said.

She stepped back. "Oh, really?"

I pulled her close again, this time easing my arms around her. "It's my significant other. He's always telling me to be gentle, and I just get so excited."

"You sorry…" She playfully pushed me away. "Don't tell me."

I looked at her deadpanned.

"Say something!" she cried.

"I'm just…"

"What?" She threw her hands up in the air.

I stepped forward and took her hands in mine, a big smile on my face. I eased my arms around her waist. "I haven't felt this good in a long, long time. I'm still trying to get over the shock of someone wanting to spend time with me. I've been alone for so long."

"I know, I know…"

We held each other in the El Chico parking lot, not wanting to say good night, yet too afraid to end the evening any other way.

chapter thirteen

"YOU'RE LOOKING CHIPPER THIS MORNING," said Ray, one of our manic midnight staff. "You either laid one on or..."

"Or what?" I fired back, bleary-eyed from the late night mating rituals of exotic birds on Animal Planet, not to mention ESPN classics about a legendary Boston Celtic by the name of Bird.

"Never mind," he teased. "We won't go there."

I headed straight for the coffee. "You're a wise man, Ray," I said, "and a good one too." I tipped my cup, thanking him for the freshly made brew. "Anybody waiting in the ER?"

"No, but a nursing home's been calling."

"This early?" I mumbled. I glanced over the census sheet. "Man, we got beds everywhere. Could be a long day."

"Their director of nursing called back about ten minutes ago," he said, "demanding to ship this 82-year-old guy without an accepting doc or anything."

I refilled my Styrofoam cup. "They don't have a clue about criteria for admission," I said. "All they know is that their 80-year-old patient is refusing to eat and throwing a temper tantrum, so he must need to be hospitalized."

"Glad I don't deal with them," he said as he opened the office door. "Too pushy for me. Hope you don't mind following up. I wasn't sure what to tell them."

"That's fine. Get out while you can before we get slammed."

My prediction came to pass, the onslaught starting early. By ten, I had three waiting in the ER and an overdose on ICU whose attending doc was demanding that the patient be transferred to psych immediately.

"Where have you been?" Carol asked as she hustled towards the ER.

"Up on ICU," I said with a smile. "Where are you going?"

"To see one of those drunks that you promised me last night."

"See, my word is gold around here," I teased, looking her up and down from a safe distance.

"It's not here that I care about," she said, glancing back at the last minute to see if I was still eyeballing her.

I was. As it turned out, someone else was watching me from the other end of the hallway.

"Hey Michael!" A familiar voice bellowed.

I turned and saw John and Maggie strolling arm-in-arm towards me. They waved, as did another shapely woman walking beside them. I froze momentarily, unable to take my eyes off of her. Embarrassed, I walked towards them, unable to wipe the schoolboy grin off my face.

"Maggie…" I smiled, extending my hand to greet her. "You actually came back to pick him up?" I slapped John on the back. "I thought you'd just leave him here for the dogs."

John bear-hugged me in return. "You'd need an army to hold me in this prison another day."

Maggie grabbed my hand. "Michael, I'd like you to meet our daughter, Jenny."

"Nice to meet you Jenny," I said with a smile, extending my hand.

She held my hand and my gaze. "From what my parents have told me, the pleasure's all mine." She gently released my hand. "I'm grateful for all you've done for them."

"Been my pleasure," I said, admiring her high cheekbones, auburn hair and glistening blue eyes. As first impressions go, she reeked of that rare combination — classy yet down to earth, cosmopolitan looks with a country girl smile. "I'm going to miss talking baseball with your dad," I turned towards John, "although he's still way off base when it comes to Mays versus DiMaggio."

"We'll have to continue that discussion over one of Maggie's home cooked meals," he said.

"Sounds good," I said, winking at Maggie just as Carol breezed by. "But it might take several dinners before we come to an agreement."

Jenny turned to her mother and smiled. "Smart man."

"I wouldn't go that far," John fired back, laughing as he squeezed my arm.

"You're off work Thursday aren't you?" Maggie asked.

"Yes ma'am," I replied, fighting back the urge to stare at her gorgeous daughter.

"Then, we'll see you Thursday," Maggie said as she grabbed John's arm and headed towards the exit.

"Looking forward to it," I said, savoring another home-cooked meal.

Jenny's eyes met mine as she turned to walk away. "Me too."

John was ecstatic, laughing and patting Maggie's hand as he reached the automatic doors leading to his freedom. Jenny glanced back and waved.

"Hey!" Carol snapped, looming in the ER doorway only a few feet away. "We need some help if you're done." She disappeared down the hallway, not giving me a chance to respond.

"Yeah, I'm done," I muttered, wondering how long she'd been

standing there. Wondering, what difference did it make? What difference should it make? One kiss last night, and suddenly she's in charge of who I talk to? Who does she think she is?

I hustled down the ER hallway and slid out the ambulance entrance, craving some fresh air and perspective before venturing back in. I leaned against the concrete pillar, my thoughts drifting. Some woman I know little about makes eyes at me and I'm gaga for her? I did her parents a good deed, and she's thanking me for that. Nothing more. Besides, up until five minutes ago I couldn't wait to see Carol. I couldn't stop thinking about her all night long. Last night was the highlight of my life over the past three years, and it wasn't the cheap margaritas. She was easy to talk to, exciting, interesting. Sexy. I imagined her in the early morning light painting in nothing more than her briefs. Her touch, her kiss… Yes, it was physical, but it was much more than that. Carol and I connected. We were old school, born and bred in the mental health wars of long ago. We were comfortable with each other.

"Why now?" I muttered as a stray cat roamed the front parking lot. Why this other woman with her sophisticated style and schoolgirl smile? Why did she intrigue me so? I was destined to find out in two days. Meanwhile, duty called.

I strolled back into the office. "What's up?"

Carol bolted by me without saying a word while David, on the phone with another nursing home, pointed to the board. We had another patient waiting to be seen and the ER doc demanding that we push the case to the forefront.

"What?" I motioned to David, who was still on the phone.

He placed the caller on hold. "What'd you do to her?"

"What's that supposed to mean?" I snapped.

"Hey, chill out, man," he said. "I'm on your side, remember?" He clicked back to the referral source.

"Sorry," I whispered as the other two phone lines lit up, triggering an onslaught of both phone referrals and walk-ins.

The afternoon was a blur, the ER exploding with three more overdose victims, one of whom died before we had a chance to assess her. She was only twenty-three years old. An eerie silence filled the ER hallway as the parents of the deceased wailed behind closed doors.

As dusk turned to darkness, I was back in the office preparing to call it a day.

"Carol still not back yet?" I asked David.

"She ran off campus for a bite to eat."

I grabbed my backpack and opened the door. "She say where she was going?"

"Nope. What's going on with her today anyway?"

"PMS I guess," I said, angry that she'd left without saying good night to me.

"Something you ain't tellin me?" he asked, the smirk on his face highly indicative of a prior conversation between the two of them.

"Nope," I smiled and headed out the door. "See ya."

"Anything you want me to pass on to Carol?" he hollered down the hall at me.

I waved good-bye and kept walking, never turning back.

chapter fourteen

"HELLO MAGGIE," I SAID WITH a smile, standing on their front porch.

"Michael!" She gave me a hug. "We're so glad you could make it."

"You kidding? I wouldn't miss one of your meals for anything."

"Still charming my mother, are you?" Jenny teased as I entered.

"Hello," I shyly replied, unable to sustain eye contact, her stunning smile catching me off guard again.

"Nice to see you again." She took my hand. "Daddy's so excited about you coming out." She led me through the formal dining room towards the den, her hand gently holding mine. "Daddy, we found him out in the street. Can we keep him?"

John crawled out of his lounge chair. "Michael, how are you?" He firmly shook my hand. He was not the same man I'd assessed a week ago. That John Robert Dalton was an angry, confused, deranged man who took a swing at me in the seclusion room and fifteen minutes later couldn't remember who I was or what he'd done.

"I'm fine," I stepped back, surprised at how relaxed I felt.

They felt like family. Like my family felt when I was growing up. Like I'd vowed to make my own family feel but failed. A sad twist of fate — repeating with my own son the one flaw of my father that haunted me so as a child — aloofness. An unexpected surge of emotion hit me.

"You okay?" Maggie asked.

"Yes ma'am." I smiled at her before turning my attention back to John. "You look great!" I patted him on the shoulder, all the while trying to keep a lid on the myriad of memories flooding me unexpectedly.

"I feel great!" John said. "Nothing like home and family to get me going again. Have a seat."

I sat down on the couch as John eased back into his La-Z-Boy. The women in his life served appetizers and drinks while we continued our discussion about America's pastime and the great players from a generation ago. From Ted Williams to Jackie Robinson and back to the iron man himself, Lou Gehrig, John gave me the lowdown on all the great names that Pop used to toss around on a lazy Sunday afternoon. It was the one time I felt close to my father.

"Real men..." John leaned forward with fire in his eyes. "Men who stood for something — integrity, honesty, commitment and guts. These men transcended their sport. An entire generation looked up to them with pride and said, 'I hope my kid grows up to be like one of them.' Name me one ball player today who can stand up to the heroes I grew up admiring."

I didn't argue with him, opting instead to listen to the ramblings of one old man lost in another time and space. Listening and wondering — Was that what old age was all about? Trying to convince the younger generation that their so-called stars of today couldn't carry the jock straps of the heroes from the past? Maybe they couldn't, I don't know. Then again, perhaps the heart of the matter had little to do with who was the greatest and everything to do with fathers and sons reliving and rejoicing in such treasures of time before the cruelty of old age erased those memories from the easels of their minds.

He leaned back in his chair, grinning from ear to ear. "I know what you're thinking.""And…" I baited him, wondering if he was truly that perceptive, hoping he wasn't reading my mind when it came to his lovely daughter, who smiled as she refilled our tea glasses.

"You're thinking I'm just some old coot who doesn't understand today's world. Well, you're right!" he exclaimed. "I don't understand why half the marriages fail and twelve-year-old kids are toting guns and drugs to school.

I nodded my head and sipped my tea.

"You know why all this is happening?" John said.

"Why?" I asked, knowing I'd hear his answer whether I wanted to or not.

"Nobody's minding the store!"

"The store?"

"The family. The kids. Everybody's out working so they can have a big screen, a fancy car and a facelift. Your me-me-me generation has built mansions to live in, yet mom and pop both work sixty hour weeks just to pay for their earthly kingdoms and all the trappings."

"Now wait a minute," I challenged, "you worked full-time at the local newspaper and ran a printing business on the side. How many hours a week was that?"

"Sometimes seventy or more," he said, "but Maggie was home taking care of the kids, and I never missed supper! I set up my printing shop out back and worked long after the kids had gone to bed." He took a deep breath and a large gulp of tea. "Now I have to admit my oldest son and I don't see eye-to-eye, but he was raised right and has turned out to be a good family man and a successful lawyer. Regardless of our differences, all that didn't happen by accident."

"Can't argue with that," I replied, my life flashing before me — the days and nights gone from family as my climb up the corporate ladder became my mistress.

"You guys done in there?" Jenny hollered from the kitchen. "We're ready to eat."

"Now that's worth fighting for," I said.

"What's that?" John stood up, stretching his legs.

"Maggie's cooking. I can see why you never missed a supper."

"You got that right!"

After supper, I tried to help out in the kitchen clean-up, but Maggie would have no part of it. Neither would John, ordering me to join him in the den. It was the Braves and Reds in Cincy, the queen city's Great American Ballpark a far cry from Crosley Field.

"That was one fine meal." I leaned back on the couch, "And chocolate pie — I can't remember the last time I ate homemade chocolate pie. I'm stuffed!"

"Glad you enjoyed it," Maggie said with a warm smile. "Now…" She reached for John's hand. "It's time for us old folk to call it a night."

"We'll continue our discussion another time," John said.

"Sounds good to me," I replied, struggling to stand, my belly stuffed. "I appreciate ya'll having me out. I'm…" I hesitated, a slight quiver in my voice, "I'm grateful." I reached out and hugged both of them, Maggie's eyes meeting mine.

"You're a good man, Michael," she whispered, letting go of me and grabbing her man of fifty-six years. "C'mon Pops!" She led him towards the hallway, glancing back with a gleam in her eye. "I got a surprise for ya."

"Oh yeah?" John put his arm around her. "I got one for you!

Remember that experimental drug they put me on?" he said with a wink. "It works!"

"Good night you two," Maggie said. "C'mon you old coot." She playfully whacked his backside and ushered him down the hallway. "Love you Jenny," her voice echoed down the hall.

"Love you too, Mom." Jenny replied, smiling at me as she gathered the cups from the table. "You want another cup, or some hot tea?"

"Coffee sounds good," I said, following her to the kitchen, feeling like a tongue-tied schoolboy alone with the girl of his dreams, wondering what to say. For a guy who had basically written off females, I was now face-to-face with a beautiful woman for the second time in a week. At least I knew Carol. We'd worked together and been friends for almost a year. We spoke the same language. Jenny, on the other hand, was a mystery. Granted, an easy-on-the-eyes, easy-to-talk-to mystery thus far, but that was with her folks around.

Alone was a different story.

chapter fifteen

"I've got something to show you," Jenny said as she flipped the kitchen lights off and headed towards the back door. I followed, spellbound as our cozy den gave way to a pitch-black deck.

I walked over to the edge. "Maggie wasn't kidding."

She joined me near the steps leading out into the yard. "About?" She spoke softly, moving ever closer to me.

"The view." I gazed skyward, awe-struck by the infinite number of shimmering stars on a moonless night. "You just don't see this in the city."

"There's a lot you don't see in the city," she said, motioning me to join her in the lounge chairs.

"So you live in the Great Smoky Mountains?" I asked, easing down into my chair.

"More like a small valley near the foothills."

"You got running water and stuff?" I teased.

"Oh, I have all the trappings," she said, "but I also have a backyard with a view. She adjusted her chair to lay back. "Don't get me wrong. I love the conveniences of home as much as anyone, but I also cherish the opportunity to turn everything off and let nature entertain for awhile."

I eased my chair back flat, the silence and sheer magnitude of the moment invigorating.

"It restores my faith in something far greater than my little world," Jenny continued, turning slightly my way. "Seems the older I get, the more I need to know God is still out there and calling the shots."

"Know that feeling all too well," I said, spellbound by the streaking light show above. "Whoa!" I tapped her forearm and pointed. "Did you see that one?"

"You are a city boy aren't you," she mused.

"Funny..." I turned towards her, warmth filling my chest. "What's that?"

"I still remember the first time I saw a rooster. I was with my mom. Four, maybe five years old. We visited a lady from the church that lived out in the country. I got so excited seeing all the animals, especially the rooster." I smiled, surprised that I could still visualize the moment. "When my dad got home from work later that day, I told him I'd seen an oyster."

"An oyster?" Jenny cackled.

"Yeah, Mom always thought I couldn't say rooster, but I'm not so convinced."

"Meaning?" she said, pulling her chair up and leaning my way.

"I'd seen cows and horses before, but that was driving down the road." I pulled my chair up to match hers. "The only books I read growing up were sports books, that and the daily newspaper. I'm not so sure that I knew the difference between a rooster and an oyster."

"So what is the difference?" she playfully asked.

"One's an aphrodisiac, and the other will make you forget about your manhood if it spurs you, or so I'm told. Or is that a goat?"

"Definitely a city slicker," she teased.

We sat in silence, the fear of being alone with this woman waning as a series of shooting stars streaked across the illuminated sky. I was still wondering what I'd done to deserve the company of two beautiful women in one week.

Jenny broke the silence. "Your folks still around?"

"Pop died sixteen years ago, rather young for today's standards."

"How old was he?"

"Sixty-four. Had a massive heart attack. Died at work."

"And your mom?" she asked.

"Still living in the house I grew up in. She's slowly fading..." I stopped, thoughts of guilt and sadness surfacing. Guilt for having left her to move to Nashville. Sadness for knowing she was all alone at night. "Thank God for my brothers," I said. "They check in on her every day."

"Were you close to your family?" she asked.

Even the darkness couldn't hide the sorrow I felt as I told her of my distant relationship with my dad and how I perpetuated the problem with my own son.

"Sad that families can't resolve old wounds and be close," she said. "I just hope my big brother, Matthew, and Daddy come to their senses before it's too late."

"Your Mom said the same thing. I feel for her. She's the one who's endured the crossfire for years."

She sat up. "Mom told you that?"

"Yeah, she..." I stopped.

She reached over and touched my hand. "It's okay. I'm not asking you to share some family secret. Mom's told me that their marriage almost fell apart at one point because of it." She slowly pulled her hand back, the electric charge raging through my veins grinding to a halt. She eased back in her chair. "Now, she looks back and laughs about that trip to California, 'by myself', as she likes to say, to see Matthew, but at the time, it was not a laughing matter."

I turned and smiled, unable to hold her gaze, feeling like I was back in junior high and visiting my girlfriend, yearning for her parents to leave us alone, yet frightened of what might follow, much less what I was supposed to do.

"They haven't been apart since," she said, "but you know, it still eats at her some nights. She wants more than anything for the two of them to come to terms before..."

I leaned back in my chair, wondering what it would take to bring John and his estranged son together. Wondering about my long lost son.

She turned towards me. "Can I ask you a question?"

"Sure." I turned her way, taken back to be so close to her striking face.

"Does Daddy have Alzheimer's?"

"I honestly don't know." I looked away, sensing the fear in her eyes. "It's hard to distinguish Alzheimer's from just plain growing old, at least in the early stages." I turned towards her. "I've been in mental health for a long time, but it's only been in the past two years that I've come face-to-face with Alzheimer's and the elderly." I leaned back and took a deep breath. "Even though I see it every day, I'm clueless and then again amazed with the elderly couples I assess."

"How so?" she asked, her voice softening again.

"How they cope and manage and move forward on a daily basis, yet knowing, at those deepest darkest times when lying in bed unable to sleep, that the spouse they've loved, endured, cherished, despised, you name it." I gestured. "Some do fine throughout the day and turn into monsters at night, only to wake up the next morning wondering what the fuss was all about." I took a deep breath and sat back in my chair. "Spouses like your mom are forced to watch while their proud husbands, many battle-tested Army vets, are committed to geriatric psychiatric units and doctors you don't know and don't like from first impressions telling you that he needs a cocktail of medications with god-awful side effects to make him better."

We sat in silence as a cool breeze brought a chill to the air. I wanted to share with her my impression of Dr. Qualls — that he was bipolar and probably on more meds than her father — but refrained, not wanting to scare her.

Dr. Baxter was another story. I hadn't seen much of the million-dollar man around Faith General of late. The latest line had him lying low since the death of one of his research subjects. The official cause of death was listed as a heart attack, however the rumor mill ran rampant. From Baxter's experimental drug killing the old man to Qualls ordering a medication combination that blew his heart out, the hospital gossip gang wouldn't let this one die.

She turned my way, easing closer to me. "Do you know anything about the medication that Daddy's taking?"

"Not really," I said, yearning to lean into her. "As part of the research project, no one supposedly knows whether he's on the experimental drug or a placebo."

She reached up and touched my forearm. "It's been a long time since college."

I froze, ever cognizant of her closeness. "One way to determine if an experimental drug is effective," I said, easing back in my chair, "is to give half the group the experimental drug while the other half gets what's called a placebo, in essence, a sugar pill."

"Sugar pill?"

"It has no therapeutic value," I said. "They'll run a battery of tests on both groups to see if the experimental drug is working."

"So we honestly don't know if he's on it?"

"If the research is on the up and up," I said, "then no one supposedly knows which patients are on the experimental drug."

"You sound skeptical," Jenny replied as she leaned forward, her elbows on her knees, looking at me with that sophisticated yet shy, school-girl face.

"Obviously, without research, we wouldn't be where we are today with medicines."

"But?" she said, tapping me on the leg.

I looked at her and sighed.

She smiled at me. "I know you can't tell me the real scoop, but..."

"But what?" I asked, eager to please her.

"Do you think Daddy's on the experimental drug?"

"I don't know," I said. "I do know he's not the same man I interviewed a week ago."

"If he's on the experimental drug, and it's helping," she asked with the innocence of a child, "will he be able to stay on it after the research project is over?"

"I would assume so," I said. "The folks conducting the research need long term data on how patients are responding to the medication."

"You say the folks conducting the research..." She settled back in her lounge chair. "Who are they?"

"Dr. Baxter and the pharmaceutical company he either works for or represents. Sun Biotechnical is the name."

"Look!" She grabbed my arm and pointed skyward.

I turned just in time to see a large shooting star flare across the sky. "Unbelievable." I turned back towards her and smiled, boldly holding my gaze, only to freeze inside again. "What did you? Oh, the researchers, right?" I nervously turned away.

"Mom didn't care much for Dr. Baxter," she said, gracefully overlooking my angst.

"Yeah, well…" I leaned back in my lounge chair. "There's a long line of folks."

"Why's that?"

"Too arrogant for my blood," I said, "but I have no idea what kind of doctor he is."

"Or researcher?" she asked.

"Not a clue. Although…" I mused, glancing her way.

"What?" she asked, playfully kicking me.

"It's not him per say," I said. "It's the thought of research." She sat up again. "Go on."

"Like I said earlier," I raised my chair all the way up, "we can't live without it. Yet, I can't help but think about the money involved."

"That we spend on research?"

"That the winner stands to make," I replied. "How many billions have the makers of Viagra made because they were first?"

"Yeah, well, that goes to show you how sick society is."

"About?"

"The male brain," she teased, reaching across and whacking me with her left hand. "Or lack of one!" she cried. "So you invent a miracle drug that…" She started laughing.

"What's so funny?" I asked, countering her left with a right jab to her ribs.

"An eighty-year-old man on Viagra!" she cackled. "No wonder the nursing homes are out of control."

"Your mother would die if she heard such language," I teased.

"No, mother would die if Daddy…" she laughed, stood up and stretched. "Leave it to the male ego to mass produce a wonder pill for the penis while millions are starving."

I crawled out of the lounge chair and stood beside her. "Hard to argue with that."

She bumped me with her shoulder. "Pretty quick for a city

boy," she said, grabbing my hand. "Think you can handle a little country girl surprise?"

"I..." That's all I could muster, my heart suddenly racing, the adrenaline roaring through my body.

"You're blushing city boy," she teased as she led me down the steps. "C'mon!" She took off running across the yard towards the pitch-black woods just beyond Maggie's garden.

"Hey!" I shouted. "Slow down! I can't see out here."

"Okay, okay..." She stopped.

I caught up to her, breathing like a middle-aged man who'd devoured far too many Twinkies. "You're not going to..."

Before I could finish, she grabbed my hand again and led me into the woods. We stopped under a giant oak tree, the blackness of night and silence of the woods eerie yet exhilarating.

"You okay?"

"Never felt better," I lied.

"Good," she said. "Now, follow me." She turned and started climbing.

"What the..." I looked up and saw the ladder-like boards nailed into the tree.

Jenny was ten feet up and still climbing. "You coming?" she called out.

"Do I have a choice?"

She climbed ever higher into the darkness of the massive tree. "Hurry up!"

I scurried up the tree, clinging to its massive trunk, frightened by what lie above, terrified of what might take a bite out of me below.

"C'mon!" she called out.

"Whoa!" I hadn't bothered to look up I was so focused on not falling. "What in the world?"

"Watch that last step." She grabbed my hand, hoisting me into her hideaway — a huge tree house smack dab in the middle of what I hoped was the sturdiest oak tree in the Dalton family forest. With built-in benches and shelves, an old Coleman ice chest and a vintage lantern, it was the finest tree house I'd ever been in. Truth be known, it was the only tree house I'd ever inhabited.

She snatched several candles and a bottle of wine from the chest. In the flick of a Bic, our oak house in the sky was transformed into a penthouse paradise. "What do you think?"

"Holiday Inn it ain't." I replied. I did the honors on the bottle while she grabbed two glasses and several cushions packed away underneath the built-in bench. "When was the last time you were up here?" I asked.

"This morning," she said, a sheepish grin on her face as she arranged the cushions and candles. "When Mom went to bed last night, I got the urge to pay my old stomping grounds a visit."

I handed her a glass of wine. "You were out here by yourself last night?"

She sat Indian-legged on one of the cushions, her deep blue eyes dancing in the flickering candlelight. "Till three in the morning."

I eased down on my knees across from her and tasted my wine. "I can understand why," I said, turning to admire the view across the treetops like no other I'd ever experienced. "This is unbelievable."

"Beats any penthouse I've seen," she said, her soft voice enticing, her gaze reflective of a middle-aged woman who'd survived tough times and maintained her dignity and class along the way, not to mention her looks.

"Did John build this for you?" I asked.

"For me and Matthew," she said. "Daddy and our favorite uncle. 'Bout killed themselves doing it. Mom worried herself sick."

"How old were you?"

"Seven. Matthew was fourteen. We thought we ruled the world from up here. My only problem was getting big brother to share it with me."

I scooted up on my knees. "You ever talk to him?"

"We've grown close in the past four to five years," she said, "cyberspace close. He's doing well for himself, fighting white-collar crime as some type of watchdog lawyer. "Figures..." she mused. "He's been fighting Daddy and all that he stood for since the day he declared himself a conscientious objector and defected to Canada."

"That still eats away at John doesn't it?"

"It does." she nodded, a sad smile on her face. "Want some more?" She grabbed the bottle and poured. "I promise not to get you drunk and take advantage of you."

"You always keep your promises?"

"Most of the time," she fired back in her best southern belle accent. "We do aim to please."

I stood to stretch my legs. "I ain't touchin' that one."

"So tell me..." She waited on me to sit back down. "What's it like working in a psychiatric ER?"

"If someone had told me two years ago." I nestled back onto a cushion and sipped my wine. "On one hand, it's the toughest thing I've done in twenty years, and, by far, the most humbling. At the same time, I'm starting to feel better about myself."

She sat up across from me, a spitting image of what I imagined John looked at some forty years ago when he gazed into Maggie's sparkling eyes. "I understand the hard part, but how so humbling?"

"I hadn't worked the front lines in ten years," I said. "I did my blue-collar time right out of college, working my way up the mental health chain of command in my late twenties and early thirties. Since that time up until a few years ago, I'd graduated to the ivory towers, the corporate side of mental health." I sipped the wine. "I'd lost touch with my roots. Working at Faith General has definitely put me back in touch with the trenches and how tough it is day after day. Someday, if I go back to the ivory tower, I'll be a better manager for it."

"Why not go back now, if that's what you want to do?"

"I'm forty-five," I said, "I've been through one corporate downsizing, I'm too old to go through another, and too set in my ways to work for most of them, assuming they'd even want me." I took another drink. "They hire kids a lot cheaper and manipulate them to do what they want."

"I thought we were talking mental health and caring for people in need," she challenged. "You make it sound like a ruthless business."

"Trust me, it is," I said, "Psych is not the money-maker it used to be. It's tough to make a profit and run a first-rate program. That's another reason I've been humbled — seeing what the blue collars deal with every day. It's dangerous these days with the way management cuts corners with staffing."

"So why do you stay?"

"Part of it is the adrenaline rush and pulling it off, knowing I can still outwork kids half my age."

She laughed. "The male ego," she playfully held her glass up. "Gotta win the game."

"Yeah," I concede, "but thank God that side of me that needs to feel like I'm helping someone still has a heartbeat. It's been empty for too long." I filled our glasses again.

She studied my face as she drank. "So you're seeking redemption."

I looked at her, a simple question, yet one never asked of me. "Perhaps."

"Is that why you went out of your way to help my father?"

Her abruptness caught me off guard.

"That came out wrong," she gently recanted.

"It's okay," I replied.

She smiled, her eyes soft. "So why'd you do it?"

I wanted to fire back because I knew I'd get to meet their lovely daughter, but I bit my tongue and took a deep breath, pondering the heart of the matter. "Your mom touched me that day, her commitment and devotion." I stood, hoping to hide the lump in my throat. "Your folks represent my parents and a simpler place in time when a couple's commitment to each other truly meant something." I glanced at her, unable to hold a steady gaze. "I certainly failed that standard, as have most of my generation."

"Me included," she quietly replied.

"Looking into your mom's eyes the night your father was admitted, I saw the genuine hurt, the fear, and ultimately the unconditional love that she felt for your dad." I felt my voice tremble. "It just hit me, that's all." I took a deep breath and let it out.

Jenny stood up beside me, gently touching my hand. "You okay?" She gazed into my eyes, a tranquil look on her face.

"Yeah, just..." I couldn't finish, overcome with emotion.

She slowly put her arms around my neck, easing me into an embrace. I held her tight, a decade of guilt, hurt and remorse that I'd slowly stuffed away suddenly spewing while in the arms of a woman I'd barely known for a day, yet felt like I'd known for a lifetime.

"You're not a sloppy cry-in-your-wine drunk are you?" she teased.

I let out a nervous laugh. "Guess I haven't been practicing my profession, huh? Keeping old garbage bottled up for years." I pulled back momentarily, intrigued by the feel of her body next to mine. "I'm sorry."

"I haven't had a good man, or any man for that matter, cry on my shoulder in a long time."

I pulled back and wiped the tears from my eyes, apologizing again for my unexpected flood of emotions. She touched my cheek, her eyes filling with tears.

"My turn," she whispered.

I started to speak, but she touched my lips with her hand.

There we stood.

In the dead of night, a universe of stars shimmering above.

Suspended in space — a mammoth, old, oak tree graciously sharing its bough.

It was there that we gingerly held each other as the flickering candlelight danced well into the wee hours of the morn.

chapter sixteen

I CRAWLED OUT OF MY CAR and hustled to the back door, milking every free moment I could muster before succumbing to whatever madness the psychiatric winds blew our way today. I keyed the side hall entrance and opened the door, thrilled to see no patients waiting for the moment. I unlocked the office door and entered.

"Hey stranger," Carol called out. "I called the other night but..." She stopped, her point well taken.

I grinned. "Yeah, well, with my renewed sense of self, I've been getting out more."

"Maybe I can work myself into your busy schedule," she said, her tone sarcastic as she grabbed an assessment and headed for the ER. "That is, if you're still interested," she said, closing the office door. Before I knew what had hit me, the door flew open. She stuck her head in. "Or available," she teased, a warm smile on her face as she closed the door again and started down the hallway.

I reopened the door. "Oh, I'm definitely interested," I fired back, stepping into the hallway. "I'll just have to check my social calendar to see when I can fit you in."

"You know what you can do with that calendar don't you?" She fired the last shot back and kept walking.

"Yeah, yeah," I muttered as I returned to the assessment office for another day in psychiatric paradise.

As with most first days back after my four-day hiatus, my twelve-hour shift was one big blur. Like a giant revolving door, as fast as the units were discharging the patients, we had new ones showing up in the lobby. Unfortunately, our end of the revolving door was stuck as the ER backed up with both psychiatric and medical patients, all of whom were agitated about the long wait.

"What's holding up your patient going to the stress unit?" Carol snapped as we passed each other in the hall. "Can't you get him moved now? I got one going up there too."

"He's been ready for an hour," I fired back. "The unit's waiting on housekeeping to clean the room."

"Or maybe the unit's delaying admissions till after shift change, huh?"

"Imagine that," I replied. "Hey, we still on for tonight?"

"Let me check my social calendar and see," she smirked as she disappeared down the hallway.

As was becoming the rule rather than the exception, my 7 p.m. clock-out time was pushing 8 p.m. when the phone rang in the office. I was halfway out the door, hoping to hustle home and spruce up before meeting Carol at O'Charley's for a nightcap.

"I shouldn't do this," I muttered as I slammed my backpack down on the desk. Carol and David were tied up in the ER, and our evening tech was stuck on our acute unit where my last admission graciously waited to "kick somebody's ass" on the unit and not down here with me.

"Assessments, this is Michael," I left off my usual and customary, 'may I help you?' phrase, too numb to care at the moment.

"Oh, Michael, I'm so glad I caught you before you left," a frantic, yet familiar voice cried.

"Maggie? What's going on?"

"It's John," her voice quivered, "he's not doing well."

"What happened?" I sat down in the cubicle, ignoring two other phone lines ringing.

"It started the day after Jenny left. His moods are so unstable. One minute he's okay, but I'll ask him something a few minutes later, and it's as if he doesn't know what I'm talking about. I'm scared, Michael. I thought everything was going to be okay, but he's acting like he did before we put him in the hospital."

"When is he scheduled for a follow-up with his doctor?"

"That's the other thing," her voice cracking, "he was supposed to see Dr. Baxter today but refused to go."

"Baxter? Was he going to see him or Dr. Qualls?"

"Oh, it's Baxter all right," she said. "His office has called twice, Dr. Baxter himself the second time."

"What'd he say?" I asked, wondering why Baxter called and not one of his staff.

"He told me to bring him in tomorrow, and if John refused, to call and he would get the police out if necessary," she said. "I don't want the police involved again, but I don't know what to do."

"Is he still taking his medication?" I asked.

"As far as I can tell."

"What do you mean?"

"Maybe it's me, but when I asked about his medicine, he had that same coy look on his face that he always has when I know he's up to something. He's never been one to take medications anyway. What should I do?"

"Where is he right now?" I asked, waving to Carol as she entered the office.

"He's in the den watching TV. He's okay right now."

"Do you want me to talk to him?"

"No, well, I don't know. I don't want to upset him again tonight if I can help it."

"If you need anything tonight, you call me, okay?" I said to Maggie as I smiled at Carol. "I'll be out for awhile, but let me give you my cell phone number. You call if you need anything, no matter what time."

"Thank-you Michael. I'm sorry to bother you. I just didn't know what to do."

"You did the right thing," I assured her as I signaled to Carol that I was ready to go. "You call if you need anything."

"I will. And Michael, my daughter told me that she sure enjoyed your company the other night."

"I appreciate that." I shrugged my shoulders for Carol's benefit, embarrassed by Maggie's comment, yet titillated thinking about Jenny. "You ready?" I motioned to Carol. "I can skip running home if you want to go now."

"Doing a little private counseling on the side?" she chided.

"Let's go." I grabbed my backpack one more time as David entered.

"What? You taking the fifth on that question?" she teased.

"I'm gonna need a fifth if I don't get outta here."

⤞

"What was that call all about?" Carol inquired as we settled into our booth at O'Charley's.

"Maggie." I glanced at the menu. "John's symptoms are back."

"What did she expect?"

"A miracle," I said, "like every other family member who wants a loved one and their lives to go back to the way it was." I flipped the menu over. "Are we eating or binging on desserts?"

She slid her menu off to the side. "Desserts sound good to me." She playfully flipped my menu. "So what's this miracle you're referring to?"

"We see families on the front end, at their lowest moment,"

I said as I stashed my menu on top of hers. "It's different after they've been treated and go home."

She ordered chocolate cheesecake, flirting with the college-aged male waiter before turning back to me. "I'm with you."

"You sure?"

She kicked me under the table. "Testy tonight, are we?" She gave me a sarcastic smile. "So what happens when the miracle fails?"

"You start with a dose of faith that the doctors and the program can help."

"Okay..." She sipped her Bailey's and coffee.

"When your loved one comes home and is doing well," I said, "your faith transforms into hope. Hope that things may, indeed, go back to the good ol' days."

"And?" Her face lit up at the sight of chocolate cheese cake.

"The part we don't see," I continued, "even though we know it happens all the time." I reached across the table with my fork, aiming towards her prize.

"I don't think so," she said, defending her treat.

"Not even a nibble?" I pleaded. She supervised while I was allowed one small bite. "Hmm... As good as it gets." I grinned.

"That's all you're getting," she said, a seductive smile on her face. "Now finish your story. Your patient returns home and everybody's feeling good."

"Hope," I said, digging into my chocolate brownie smothered in ice cream.

"The patient deteriorates, sometimes even worse," she said, "and all that faith and hope go out the window. Then what?"

"I think Paul, a great man of God, said it best. 'And now these three remain: faith, hope and love. But the greatest of these is love'." I grabbed the coffee pot and filled our cups. "I never realized how tough that roller coaster ride was on the families until tonight when Maggie called."

"How so?"

"That tone in her voice," I said, reaching for the sugar to sweeten my coffee, "the fear, and then anger at both John and the doctors, the anguish that follows such a devastating letdown." I stirred two packs into my cup of java. "All she's got left is the love. That's all that will get her through."

"So what's she gonna do?"

"Try to get him to the doctor tomorrow. He was supposed to go today, but refused.

What I can't figure out is why he was scheduled to see Baxter instead of Qualls."

"Meaning?"

"Maggie said that Baxter actually called their house, upset that John had missed his appointment. Go figure." I took a heaping bite of my brownie and snuck a bite of her crust.

"Faith General's anointed one?" Carol said.

I placed the money for our treats on the table. "Baxter conducting follow-up calls?"

"Hard to believe he'd waste his time on a patient receiving the placebo."

"Who knows," I replied, finishing off my dessert. "I thought no one, including the attending docs, knew who got the placebo and who got the supposed miracle vaccine."

She swallowed her last bite. "Possibly the same vaccine that killed the other patient."

"Whatever happened with that investigation?" I asked.

"Outside of the rumor mill, no one's talking."

"Makes you wonder." I thanked the waiter and glanced at Carol, wondering what was next. I didn't have to wait long for an answer.

She looked me straight in the eye. "My place or yours?"

"Ah..." I quickly looked down.

"You're blushing again," she said as she touched my hand,

that charged feeling shooting through my veins. "Follow me home for a nightcap." She smiled mischievously. "Unless, of course, your social calendar or community status has suddenly changed in the past four days."

"No," I grinned. "I believe I'm available, but I should call my secretary to make sure."

"You just might need a legal secretary by the time I'm done with you."

chapter seventeen

IT WAS NINE IN THE morning, and all was quiet on the psychiatric front. The onslaught of patients continued long after I'd left work last night, leaving us no room at the psychiatric inn to start this day. With David running late and Carol not due in for another hour, I kicked back in the office, pinching myself to see if the events of the past week were real, or was I waking up from a very pleasant dream. My pinch came in the form of an unexpected cell phone buzz.

"Michael?" The troubled voice was unmistakable.

"Maggie, what's going on?" I asked.

"It's John. He chased the nurse from our house."

"Nurse? What nurse?" I dropped my feet from the desk. "Maggie, are you okay?"

"No," she replied, her voice cracking.

"Did he hurt you?"

"Oh no! He didn't do anything to me."

"Where is he right now?"

"By the front door, watching out for her."

"Her who?" I asked, abruptly standing, silently thinking, *I can't even muster five measly minutes to kick back.*

"That nurse," Maggie blurted out. "He thinks she's trying to poison him."

"Who sent a nurse out to your house?"

"I don't know," she frantically replied. "I think your hospital sent her."

"What? I don't understand. What'd she say?" I asked.

"Something about following up since John couldn't make it in to see the doctor."

"Was she from Dr. Baxter's office?" I asked as another phone line rang. "Maggie, can you hold a second. I've got to grab this other line. I'll be right back, okay?" I snatched the receiver and was confronted with a drugged-out whiny female.

"Don't you wanna hear what I gotta say?" she slurred.

"We're not a phone counseling service and all our units are full. Check back with us late this afternoon, or I'll be glad to give you the number to several other programs."

"I'll just take all these pills and kill myself," she snapped.

I recognized her voice from yesterday. She'd called four times, demanding that we send a taxi to the Dickerson Road dive where she was holed up. I gave my usual spiel about her safety and getting to the nearest emergency room, offering in the process to call #911.

Click.

"Thank you," I muttered as I hung the receiver up, grabbed my cell phone, and clicked back to Maggie.

"Maggie?" I said a second time.

She was gone.

I started to dial, but didn't know her number. I checked my cell phone but was clueless as to how to retrieve the number. "That's what you get, idiot," I murmured, angry that I still hadn't taken the time to manipulate my phone beyond simply answering it or dialing a number. I stuffed my cell phone back in my pants pocket, pulled up John's demographic information on my computer, and frantically dialed their home number. It immediately kicked to voice mail.

I wasn't sure what to do. I felt helpless, knowing I couldn't leave until David showed up. Knowing I shouldn't leave. I wasn't obligated to John and Maggie, or, for that matter, Jenny, their beautiful daughter. Why risk my job for them? I dialed their number again. It kicked over to voice mail as before. I started to dial the police but hesitated, given what transpired the last time they were called out to Maggie and John's home.

"C'mon David," I mumbled aloud, pacing like a caged animal. Most days, his tardiness was annoying but not earth shattering. This morning, however, was a different story. I had no way of knowing what was happening. Had John pulled the phone chord out of the wall in a fit of rage? Was he out of his mind and going after Maggie again? Or was it something simple like a call waiting glitch? Surely Maggie would call right back. I couldn't bring myself to dwell on the worst case scenario, knowing that if, indeed, John was in a delusional state and going after Maggie and I chose not to call the police…

"Good morning!" David cried in his usual, happy-go-lucky, never-mind- that-I'm-twenty-minutes-late self. "Are we busy?"

"Just a call or two," I said. "We're out of beds."

He went straight to the coffee pot. "Until mid-morning when the docs make rounds."

I grabbed my backpack. "While it's quiet, I got a favor to ask."

"Shoot."

"I need to run off campus for about an hour, maybe two. Can you handle it?"

"Yeah, sure, Carol will be in soon. If four or five show up in the lobby, they can wait," he said, hinting that I needed to hurry back. "What's up?"

"It's a long story, but do me a big favor," I replied, already halfway out the door.

"Another one?"

"If a lady named Maggie calls asking for me, tell her I'm on my way. If she doesn't need me, David, you listening?" I snapped as he seemed oblivious to what I was telling him. "Ask her if everything is okay. If things are fine and she doesn't need me to come out, please call me. That way I'll know to turn around. You got it?"

"Gotcha!" he gestured. "Get outta here."

"I'd better let Jo know. Is she in yet?"

"I saw her as I walked in," he said. "She was headed to a meeting. Text her."

"Yeah, right," I scoffed.

"You still don't know how to text?" David asked, genuinely amused.

"Think she'll be okay if I just leave her voice mail?" I asked, anxious to get on down the road.

"She'll be fine," he said. "You know Jo — easy come, easy go."

I was out the door again. "Please call if she calls and..." I was jogging down the hall.

"Yeah, yeah, just hurry back before the floodgates open."

I sped down the two-lane highway, my mind racing again. What if John's delusional and doesn't recognize me? What if he's wielding a knife? What if he's already hurt Maggie? Or himself accidentally?

On the other side of the ledger, my thoughts were reeling about work. What would my boss say if she knew I was leaving to check on a former patient? Unauthorized home visits were forbidden. And then there was Baxter. If he knew I was meddling with one of his research patients... Unless, of course, I persuaded John to return to Baxter.

I topped sixty miles-per-hour on the straight-a-ways, questioning why I stayed in a job that exposed me to every known virus spewing down the ER pike. Not a week went by that I wasn't face-to-face with an angry AIDS patient or a drugged-out hepatitis victim — as deadly as AIDS and far more prevalent. And all those times we're called to help restrain out-of-control, infected patients trying to bite, kick or scratch their way loose. And lest we forget the guy with AIDS who tried to spit in my face. Why was I doing this job? Surely by now I could find another middle-management position in healthcare and work my way back up the corporate ladder. Why stay?

As I leaned into the hairpin curves, my thoughts veered still another direction — to Jenny, to Carol, to my ex-wife and my son. What am I doing? Where am I going? I'm forty-five years old and acting like a crazed, hormone-charged teenager. If I had any sense, I'd call my ex-wife and beg her to take me back. Maybe, just maybe after four years, she'd reconcile. But for what? So I can get another corporate job and fly the friendly skies? She's not going down that path again, and frankly, neither am I. At least not with her. We had our good times, but I'm not in love with her. I'm not even in love with the memory of what we had, so why in the world was I thinking of her now?

Was I afraid of a new relationship? Afraid of commitment? Shouldn't I be? Why not have some fun while I've still got a hormone or two jumping around my soon-to-be, too-old-to-attract body? When was the last time I held two different women in the same week? Why stop with two fish when there's a wide open sea out there? I'm sure I can muster a line or two.

Even if I wanted to be committed to one, who do I set sail with? Carol's quick, witty, fun to be around, easy on the eyes and knows me pretty well. If that doesn't scare her off, then we're either made for each other, too scared to admit that opportunity rarely knocks anymore, or too delusional to know better. Jenny, in some ways, is a whole lot like Carol — strong and independent, down-to-earth, and with a flair for the artistic. She, too, was easy on the eyes, very easy. But something about her beauty transcended that gorgeous school-girl smile. Carol has it too, come to think of it. Something spiritual, ethereal.

As much as my over-the-hill body craved their touch, it was the tenderness of their hearts that attracted me so. Maybe my graying head had absorbed a bit of wisdom, I don't know. Whatever the case, I wasn't sure where I was going with the women in my life. Maybe I was the delusional one for even thinking that either one of them was that interested.

"Oh no! No!" I pounded the steering wheel as I approached their house. I parked near the street, their driveway crammed with two police cars and two other cars that I didn't recognize.

"Who are you?" one of the officers snapped.

"A friend of John and Maggie's," I replied as I opened the front screen door and entered, only to be derailed by the same cop with an attitude. He didn't look old enough to be driving, much less toting a gun in the name of the law.

He grabbed my arm. "Well, now is not the best time to be paying them a visit."

"Look," I shook loose of his hold, "I work at Faith General. I know John well. Maggie called me at the hospital this morning to come out."

To my surprise, the cop grabbed me again, only harder this time. "You didn't hear me did you? I said now is not the best time to pay them a visit, so why don't you..."

I didn't give him a chance to finish, slipping his grasp a second time as I called Maggie's name. He started after me, only to be called off by his older, more sensible partner. I scurried through the kitchen and out onto the back deck where two other policemen struggled to get handcuffs on John. Watching the cops were two unknown females, one wearing nursing scrubs, the other a young girl in jeans and a sloppy, hang down shirt.

"Michael!" Maggie cried, terrified and in tears as she grabbed my arm.

"What's going on?" I asked, hugging her with my left arm while assessing John. "John, talk to me," I said. "Are you okay?"

"And you are?" the snotty-nosed kid in blue jeans barked, holding her cellular phone in one hand and a notebook in the other.

"I'm a friend of the family," I replied as I again tried to get John's attention. The cops had him cuffed and were walking him towards the back gate. I stepped in front of them, my eyes begging to please give me a chance to connect with him. They obliged. With Maggie still by my side, I looked John right in the eye, placing my hand on his shoulder.

"John, it's Michael. Talk to me. What happened?"

"That nurse!" He turned towards the bewildered woman, who had eased her way closer to the door. "She barged in here and tried to make me take some medicine. This is our home! They don't have the right to force their way in here!"

"Easy..." I pulled him into me, whispering in his ear. "John, you know I'm on your side. Take some deep breaths and let me find out what's going on, okay? We'll figure something out. Just take it easy." I released him, again reassuring both he and Maggie.

"Can we take the cuffs off?" I asked the policeman.

"It's policy," the cop replied.

"What in the world happened here?" I asked, motioning the cops to hold their position. They remained cordial. I looked to the nurse for some answers. She, however, was not the one in charge.

The blue-jeaned stranger stepped in. "You said you were a friend of the family?"

"That's right. Who are you?" I fired back.

"Virginia," she snapped. "I'm with the mobile crisis unit."

"So why were you called out?" I countered, turning again towards the nurse, who turned back to the door, apparently still shaken.

Virginia stepped forward. "I'm not sure what your purpose for being here is, but Mr. Dalton was threatening bodily harm to her." She pointed to the nurse. "She feared for her safety, and we were called out to assess the situation."

"Maggie, what happened here?" I turned towards her.

"Excuse me," the mobile crisis worker butted in, "I've already determined what happened here, okay. I've made my disposition and the police are here to carry that involuntary committal order out. If you want to find out what happened, that's fine. But, I don't need to detain these officers any longer and..."

"Wait a minute," I demanded. No wonder John had to be restrained. I wasn't far behind him at the rate this conversation was going. Unbeknownst to the crisis worker, I dealt with mobile crisis all the time. They were one of our main referral sources for psychiatric patients, and, for the most part, performed a solid job out in the field where police back-up was often needed to ensure everyone's safety.

The scary part of the equation – an inexperienced crisis counselor could complete a measly workshop and become authorized by the state to evaluate and subsequently sign an initial set of involuntary committal papers on anyone in the community, including going into private homes.

"You've done what?" I cried out, Maggie taken back by my outburst. "A committal based on what?" I demanded, refusing to give her a chance to answer. Instead, I turned to the silent nurse to get her take on all that had transpired. "So what happened? And who do you work for?"

"I'm with Faith General's home health service," she replied.

"I've been assigned to work with Dr. Baxter and his research project."

"With or without their permission, I see," I chastised. In all fairness to her, she was caught in the middle. Baxter had sent her out following John's no-show to his office. She had no idea what she was walking into.

"Whether you agree or not," Virginia retaliated, "I've assessed him and feel he's a danger to himself or others and should be admitted to the hospital for..."

"Who gave you admitting privileges?" I interrupted, livid by now.

"I have the authority to..."

"I know all too well what authority you have," I interrupted as I walked back over to John, Maggie clinging to my arm. "Your committal paper gets him to the ER and that's all. It's up to the ER physician to decide if he's truly committable."

Realizing that I had no authority to override her decision, I explained to John and Maggie what was happening and assured them that I'd talk to the ER doctor as soon as we arrived. It saddened Maggie and sickened me that John, handcuffed like a hardened criminal, was forced into a police cruiser for the second time in the past month.

Maggie followed my car back to Faith General. Prior to leaving work, I hadn't even noticed which ER doc was on. I prayed that it was Halston. He was the only chance we had of getting John sent back home today. The other ER docs were already in Baxter's back pocket and would follow his lead to have John readmitted.

The other question burning in my mind — Why was Baxter so determined to reel John back in?

chapter eighteen

Jo, my supervisor, caught me as I entered our office. "You got a second?" She motioned for me to step out in the hallway. "I need to talk to you."

I looked at Carol, who looked at David, who looked back at Jo. From the looks on their faces, I knew I was in trouble and deeper than anticipated. Jo escorted me down the ER hallway to the grief room and closed the door. I knew what was coming.

The mobile crisis worker on the scene had put two and two together and connected me to the assessment office at Faith General. Jo was not overjoyed since mobile crisis was a key referral source. However, the damage done could be smoothed over. It was Baxter's nurse, the silent one on the scene, who caused grave concerns for me. She, too, had either recognized me or overheard Maggie mention that I worked at the hospital. She felt obliged to relay the events of the day to Baxter's office. By the time the news of my escapades went from Baxter's nurse to Baxter to the hospital CEO to Jo's boss and finally, Jo herself, I'd all but kidnapped John and held the mobile crisis worker hostage.

"You've got to back off," Jo pleaded. "Baxter's pegged you as a troublemaker who's trying to sabotage his research."

I shook my head. "That's a crock."

"I know that," she assured me, "but what I think has nothing to do with it."

I flopped into the chair and crossed my arms. "What are you telling me?"

Jo leaned forward, her eyes intense. "The CEO will bend over backwards to keep Baxter happy and the research money pouring in." She waited on me to look at her.

I took a deep breath, nodded, and exhaled, slowly releasing the disdain raging through my veins at the mention of Baxter's name.

Jo whacked me on the foot. "You know how the game is played."

"And?" I frowned, sensing her answer.

She shook her head as she pulled back.

"Bottom line?" I asked, my eyes telling her that I wasn't angry at her.

"Stay away from this case."

I nodded. "Okay."

With that, she dismissed me to the ICU to assess a 21-year-old overdose victim. I complied, but not before asking Carol to get word to Maggie that I'd been ordered to stay away.

I took the stairs up to the ICU, seething with every step at the thought of Baxter belittling me before the hospital brass, making it sound like I was interfering with his sacred research subjects. He didn't care that I'd convinced John to stay the course and work the program, or that I'd worked diligently with Maggie to ease her mind and garner her support as well. All he cared about was his research, and anybody who got in the way of his wishes was going down one way or the other.

Drained from the drama swirling around me, I decided to chill out in the ICU. Instead of my customary ten to fifteen minute interview, I sat back and talked with a 21-year-old kid who reminded me an awful lot of another boy turned man — my son. Both were troubled by the stark reality that the magical age of twenty-one had little to do with manhood. I was living proof of such. This kid, however, wound up in an ICU with a tube shoved down his throat.

As I conversed with the young man, I couldn't help but wonder what separated him from my son. His voice was hoarse and raspy as he spoke of his parents' divorce when he was still in high school. And, as karma would have it, the young man's father flew the coop and never looked back, moving to a new city and a new life, or so presumed. Still, the kid's home life appeared stable. He hadn't been abused as a child, nor had he come from a family gene pool saturated with mental illness or addictions. He was a college kid away from home who was flunking physics, questioning his commitment to an engineering degree, and falling out of love with his girlfriend. An argument with her triggered a drunken stupor and his subsequent suicide attempt as he downed a half-full bottle of Tylenol before passing out on his dorm bed.

He was genuinely embarrassed by what he'd done, yet continued to speak of feeling all alone and trapped in a life he wasn't sure he wanted anymore. When it came time to end the interview, I couldn't look him in the eye, at least not until I gathered my wits and kicked into Hollywood overdrive. Only then could I shake his hand and wish him well.

Once outside of the ICU, I took the elevators down to the basement and slipped outside on the back side of the hospital. Hidden from view, I leaned against the old building and took a long deep breath. I couldn't look into that boy's eyes for fear of seeing my son's eyes crying out to me. I shook my head in disgust, sickening thoughts of my boy and how he, too, could be severely depressed, even suicidal, and I would never know it until it was too late.

I pulled my cell phone out of my pocket, grabbed the reading glasses resting high atop my head, and called every number I had for him, leaving messages at both his dorm room and his mother's house. I wasn't sure how he would respond to my out-of-the-blue call. The last time we'd conversed was five months ago at Christmas, and that was a brief, tension-filled phone conversation. He still harbored a great deal of anger towards me, making it too easy for me to lay low, rationalizing that one day he'd find it in his heart to forgive me. However, the truth of the matter was that I'd quit trying to reach out to him. I, too, was hurt and angered that he'd sided with his mother and shut me out.

I stashed my phone back in my pants pocket and took the long way back to the ER, hoping, by chance, that I would run into Maggie. I slipped into the ER nursing station and spoke briefly with the nurses, all three of whom were preoccupied with an ambulance only two minutes out with a 60-year-old male in full cardiac arrest. As they scampered to set up Faith General's lone trauma room, I scanned the chart rack and the counter. Nothing. Not one sign of John's chart. Something wasn't right. Even though no psych patients had come through this morning, the ER was hopping with a variety of bumps and broken bones. There's no way John could have made it through the system and upstairs in the time it took me to assess the kid on ICU and call my son.

I stormed into our office, only to find it empty and the phone ringing.

"Assessments, this is Michael. May I help you?"

"Michael."

I slumped into my chair, Jenny's voice soothing my rage for the moment.

"What's going on?" she asked. "Mom just called from there

and said Daddy was re-admitted, something about they're not letting you near him or her."

"Re-admitted?" I asked.

"You didn't know?"

I shared with her the circumstances of the day, assuring her that I would call later tonight once I found out what was going on. Carol and David strolled in just as Jenny and I shared parting pleasantries.

"Where have you been?" Carol snapped.

"Me?" I fired back, refusing to turn and face her.

"Yeah…" Carol smirked. "Sounded like a desperate female on the line."

I wanted to light into her but backed off and focused on David since he was the one handling John's case. To my surprise, he was distant and unwilling to share information.

"Will someone please tell me what's going on?" I demanded.

Carol turned towards David.

David glanced at me and then back at Carol.

"C'mon guys!" I cried.

David broke the ice. "The godfather himself told me to keep you out of this case. I'm sorry, man. I didn't ask for this either."

"Baxter told you that?"

"Just five minutes ago," he replied.

"Why the rush job on John's admit?" I asked.

He looked at Carol, then back at me and shrugged.

"Did the ER doc even assess John?" I asked, looking first at David, who offered nothing, and then towards Carol. "I'll find out, one way or the other."

"Did you not hear what he just told you?" Carol snapped.

"It's okay." David motioned to her and turned towards me. "Just know that you didn't hear this from me, okay? I need this job."

He shared the circumstances surrounding John's rapid re-admission to the geri-psych unit. Armed with reports from the home health nurse and mobile crisis, Baxter called long before John's arrival and convinced the ER doc to sign the second 6404 committal on him.

"Sight unseen?" I asked.

"A breeze by, at best," David replied, motioning the three of us to move to the back of the office. "All I know is this, and then I'm leaving it alone. I was told by Jo to meet the patient in the ER, write an addendum to the old assessment, and move him upstairs as quickly as possible, that John didn't need to be medically cleared in the ER, and Baxter wanted him to be a direct admit under his name."

"Baxter told you?"

"No, Jo told me," replied David. "Said that Baxter called her personally, as did the CEO."

"You're joking?"

"Nope. When he arrived with the police, I saw him five minutes tops. He seemed fine to me. Worried about his wife, but otherwise alert and oriented with no signs of delusional thinking, no homicidal or suicidal ideation. The man seemed fine, okay? I was just following orders."

"So what about Maggie?" I asked. "What'd she say?"

David glanced at Carol again, as if afraid to go on.

"Go ahead." She sighed. "He's won't stop until he knows."

"Knows what?" I asked.

"Maggie was very upset when I told her that you had been removed from the case," David said. "She demanded to talk to Dr. Baxter, but he never showed his face. Then she asked to speak to the CEO."

"And?" I asked.

He shrugged. "She headed up towards administration, but I got the sense that she wasn't going through with her complaint."

"Why's that?"

He again glanced at Carol, who motioned him to unload.

"Her last words to me were simply, 'Please have Michael call me.'"

I smiled at David. "Thanks." I patted him on the shoulder and plopped back down in my chair, the two of them standing over me.

"You've got to let go of this case," Carol pleaded. "And I know what Jo told you because she told me to drill it into your thick head — if Baxter wants to drop the ax, she won't be able to protect you again." She touched my shoulder.

I turned to face her, dying to reach out and pull her into an embrace, to share my innermost thoughts and fears about my son and the smoldering scorn I felt towards not only Baxter's ruthlessness but the hospital white collars who cowered before him.

"We'll find out what's happening." She glanced at David, then back at me. "But let us do it. We need you here. I need you..." She touched my cheek, her eyes begging me to back off.

"But why?" I asked. "Why's Baxter so interested in one old man? It's not like John's the only guinea pig he's got."

"Meaning?" David asked.

"I heard that he's testing some miracle drug for Alzheimer's and has research studies going on in half-a-dozen hospitals or more," I said. "That's why it doesn't make sense that he's so engrossed with John."

"Maybe it's his ego," Carol replied. "He can't take someone walking out on his study. "It's a shot to his pride, and we all know he's a control freak. He's sending a message that he's in charge and no one need challenge his authority."

"Could be," I said as I stood, "but it goes much deeper than that."

"Meaning?" Carol asked.

"I don't know," I grabbed the newest referral from the fax and turned back towards her, "But you can bet I'm gonna find out."

145

chapter nineteen

WITH THE USUAL MAD RUSH of afternoon patients demanding immediate help, the remainder of the day had flown by, leaving me little time to think about John and Maggie, or my son, who hadn't returned my earlier messages. I was hoping to track him down from home later tonight.

"Home free," I mumbled to myself as I signed off of the computer and reached for my backpack.

"We still on for tonight?" asked Carol.

"Can I get a rain check?" I replied, longing to be with her, yet yearning for the solitude of home and the hope that I'd reach my son. "C'mon…" I motioned for her to follow.

"On one condition," she said as she walked with me out the office door and down the hallway towards the time clock.

"I'm listening."

"Please call me later after you talk with Maggie."

"What?" I fired back as I reached for my ID badge. "Did Jo tell you to keep tabs on me?"

She stepped back, the hallways silent for the moment. "Sometimes you can be a real jerk."

I punched the time clock and turned back towards her. "Will you walk me to the door?"

"You being a jerk again?"

"No." I put my arm around her and headed down the back hallway towards the parking lot. "Just tired."

She bumped me with her hip. "Believe it or not, I do care about you."

"Feeling's mutual."

She stopped a few feet short of the door. "Sometimes I wonder..."

We stepped outside the ER ambulance entrance. I hugged her, my weary bones suddenly alive, or delusional, trying to convince me that I was up for another late night. "Let me see how I feel after I get home," I said. "You're here for another hour or so, right?"

"Till nine," she said as an ambulance approached.

"Maybe we can meet at O'Charley's." I stepped away, still facing her.

"I'd like that."

"I'll call," I said and headed towards my car in the employee lot a mere thirty yards away.

"Please do," she replied.

I turned and waved, then strolled past a smattering of cars to reach mine. I popped the hatchback and tossed my backpack inside. As I closed it, a huddled mass appeared behind my left front end. I froze, not sure of what I'd seen and not in any great hurry to find out. I opened and closed the hatchback again, hoping the noise would shoo away any wild animal that might have wandered down from the nearby woods. I mustered the courage to walk towards the driver's side door.

"What the..." I jumped back. "John, is that you?"

"'Bout time you got here." He started to stand.

"Stay down," I snapped, glancing back, fearful of being seen. Carol was talking with the EMTs as they unloaded their patient. I opened my car door, hoping to buy some time. "How'd you get out here?" I asked in a muffled angry voice.

"You giving me a ride," John said, "or am I walking home?"

"Do what?" I cried. I cranked the engine, climbed out, and opened the driver-side rear door as if I was getting something out of the backseat. "I can't believe..."

John remained in a crouch, his hands grasping the fender, his head tilted upward, eyes locked on mine. "Maggie said you'd help if I made it out."

"And lose the only job...?" I was angry at him, yet stoked at the thought of going one up on Baxter. "Get your sorry butt in here." I said as I pulled out of the backseat. "Stay down, there are people out here." I walked back to the hatchback and opened it, hoping to hide his crawling into the back seat. I grabbed an old blanket and eased the door shut as John scrunched across the seat, mumbling under his breath. I climbed in and backed out, all the while watching Carol.

John started to rise up.

"Stay down," I said as I hit the gas and headed towards the back exit.

"Anybody see us?" he asked.

"I don't know..." I turned right and sped towards the back gate.

"What?"

"Carol started towards us," I said. "I acted like I didn't see her, but I don't think she bought it."

"Who's Carol?"

"It's a long story,"

"Are we out of the parking lot yet?"

"Yeah." I looked back in the rear view mirror one more time, wondering if this was the last time I'd be pulling out of Faith General's parking lot as an employee. "You can sit up now."

I sped towards the highway, my thoughts racing, wondering if anyone saw what just transpired. I glanced in the rear view mirror at the old man looking back and me with a big grin on his face. "How'd you break out?" I asked.

John laughed as he gingerly climbed into the front seat. "I'm an old Army man. We got our ways."

We were well beyond the hospital grounds, motoring away from Music City towards Springfield. Like two old friends, we rode in solitude, lost in the moment, wondering what tomorrow would bring.

John broke the silence as we exited the interstate for the back roads home. "I'll make this up to you," he said, patting my shoulder like a father assuring his son. As much as I appreciated his concern, I wasn't convinced the sun was coming up for me tomorrow, at least not over Faith General.

"Did anybody see us?" he asked, sensing my anguish.

"I don't think so," I replied, my eyes glued to the two-lane road that was fast becoming a familiar trek.

"What about your friend in the parking lot?"

"Carol? I don't think she saw anything."

"Would she cover for you if she did?"

I glanced his way. "Hope we don't have to find out."

John leaned back and took a deep breath. "Me too."

"Maggie know you're coming?"

He turned towards me and grinned. "What do you think?"

I laughed. "So what's next for you two? Robbing a bank!"

"You never know what we might pull off next."

"Yeah, well," I leaned in and tapped his left knee, "you know this ain't over."

"Meaning?" he asked.

I straightened back up, both hands on the wheel as we approached the last curve before their house. "Baxter," I said with contempt, knowing that he had the power to get me fired and the privileged arrogance to enjoy the moment, not to mention what he might do to John.

"What about him?" John sat up, his eyes glued to the road.

"How'd you wind up on the unit so fast?" I asked.

"What do you mean?"

"Did you even see the ER doc?"

"Not really," he said. "He stuck his head in and asked how I felt. I told him fine, and that was it."

"And what about David's assessment?" I asked.

"Assessment?" He leaned back, slightly off-balance from the sharp curve.

"Questions about your memory, what happened today, the same stuff I asked you the first time we met," I said as I eased off the gas. "Did David ask you a bunch of questions like that?"

"He told me and Maggie that he'd be working my case up, and it shouldn't take long." John leaned in, his left hand grasping my headrest. "What's your point?"

"Baxter arranged all that," I said. "He made all the calls ahead of time to make sure you'd be admitted without a hitch."

"What are you saying?" he asked.

"That for some reason, Baxter wants you back on the unit and under his control."

"But why?"

"I don't know," I said as I turned into their driveway. "I was hoping you could tell me."

"Look!" John's face lit up like a little boy seeing the lights of the state fair for the first time. He was out the door before I could even slide the gearshift into park. In a scene from an old movie, I stood by the car as two old souls held each other on their front porch, embracing as if they hadn't seen each other in fifty years.

"Michael!" Maggie motioned me to join them.

I walked over, relaxed and grateful for another opportunity to spend time with the Dalton gang.

"I just knew you'd be here." She draped her arm around me, tears welling up in her eyes. "How can I ever thank you for what you've done?"

"Simple," I said as I joined them inside. "Feed me."

"My pleasure," Maggie replied, "but first, I've got someone on hold who wants to talk to you." She grabbed the phone and handed it to me, then took John's hand and led him into the den.

"Hello." I stepped back out on the front porch, flipping the lights off.

"Sounds like you're fast becoming one of the family," Jenny said.

"For better or worse, huh?" I said as I took a deep breath of fresh country air and gazed above at the multitude of twinkling lights and a crescent moon hanging around the western sky.

"You okay?" Jenny asked.

"A little tired from all the excitement with Bonnie and Clyde."

"They're quite the twosome."

I laughed. "Like nothing I've ever seen."

"I hope Daddy's situation doesn't cause you any problems with your job."

"Me too."

"What's going to happen to him now?"

"The hospital will report him AWOL to the police since he is classified as an involuntary patient."

"Meaning?"

I sat down on the porch. "Most of the time the police simply relay the information out to paroling officers."

"That's all they'll do?"

"Depending on the condition of the patient," I said. "In John's case, the local sheriff's department will be on the lookout."

"You think they'll…" Her voice trailed off.

"It's not them I'm worried about."

"Then who is it?" she asked.

"Dr. Baxter."

"You find what you were looking for in the trunk?" chided Carol over the phone.

"Trunk?" I asked, hoping to sound surprised as I set my car keys on the coffee table and plopped down on my couch.

"At least have the decency to shoot straight with me," she fired back.

I didn't know what to say. I'd forgotten to call while at John and Maggie's. Two hours later, I heard her short and not-so-sweet message on my cell phone. I hated to call but knew I had to. She deserved better from me.

"I hope you're not involved in the great escape."

I didn't answer, not wanting to lie to her, much less involve her. I tried to smooth things over, but she wasn't buying it and I couldn't blame her for it. Our conversation ended on a sour note, leaving me to ponder whether I'd been seen driving John away from the hospital. Even though the parking lot appeared vacant, other employees were leaving at the same time. Housekeeping could have been peering out one of six floors of windows. Security...

I sank deep into the couch, a queasiness stirring in my gut. I took a rare shot of Jack Daniels, bypassing the coke mixer on my coffee table. "Just how dumb?" I scoffed, the realization smacking me in the face — the hospital parking lots were under video surveillance. "Twenty-four, seven," I muttered.

I grabbed the bottle again. "What are my odds?" I asked Mr. Daniels as I downed another shot. It wasn't every day that a geri-psych patient eloped. They were quickly found on the rare occasion one snuck out the door. Never had one made it off grounds, much less through the night.

"Then again," I mused as I cradled *my* TV buttons, "John Dalton is not your everyday geri-psych patient."

chapter twenty

I AWOKE ON MY COUCH WITH a god-awful hangover and glanced at the clock. I had fifty minutes to shave, shower and stumble into work. "Or…" I grabbed the half-empty bottle of Jack Daniel's sitting on the coffee table, my head throbbing, my gut churning, grateful that I had no desire to take an early morn swig. "Although…" I headed for the shower, sensing that the forecast for today was stormy.

I clocked in four minutes late and scampered down the back hallway, yearning for a strong cup of coffee. I walked into the assessment office and was greeted by Jo, her boss, and the chief of security for the hospital. There was only one reason for his presence.

"I'm sorry to inform you…" Jo's words faded into a flood of memories flashing before my eyes. Twenty-five years in the mental health wars, and I'd never so much as been disciplined or written up, my work ethic as blue collar as my old man's, my white-collar days as a program director impeccable. And how many middle-aged, ex-managers could make it back in the trenches, much less a psychiatric ER, as I'd done over the past two years.

"Michael." Jo tried to bring me back to reality, her sad eyes telling me that she was following orders from above. "Is there anything you want to say?"

"No." I gave her a hug. "You're good people, Jo," I whispered. "Thanks for the opportunity."

"Why'd you do it?" asked Clint, the head of security and a man I respected.

I stood and swallowed hard as the butterflies fluttered in my belly. I looked up at Clint and anchored myself on the back of my chair. "I always strived to treat patients as I'd want my family treated," I said, easing over to the door, taking one last look around the office. "When I look at this particular case and these two people…" I cleared my throat, fighting to keep it together, "I'd want somebody to rescue my father or grandfather under the same circumstances." I started to walk out but stopped. "It's sad this hospital's sold out to a doctor they don't even know."

"What's that supposed to mean?" Jo's boss barked. He'd stood there the entire time, stone-faced, not uttering one word. Since I'd just been fired, I had no reason to worry about repercussions from the ivory tower.

"You think Baxter is in this for the good of this hospital?" I said. "You think he genuinely care about his patients?" I caught my breath and reloaded, my passion trumping my nerves. "He's after one thing and one thing only. He wants to win the research race and doesn't care who he tramples in the process."

"What race?" he asked.

He was either dumber than I'd initially given him credit for in regards to the billion dollar race for an Alzheimer's vaccine, or shrewd enough to wonder what I was thinking since I represented opposing forces. At this point, I didn't really care. I was just glad that he'd opened the door for me to take a parting shot.

"Don't you ever wonder why an Ivy League doctor wound up at Faith General as opposed to Vanderbilt or St. Thomas?" I said. "There's a skeleton in his closet somewhere."

Clint afforded me one last look around the ER on my way out the door. As much as the blue-collar pay was a bitter pill to swallow, I'd grown to love this job. It was an adrenaline rush at times, juggling multiple cases simultaneously, not to mention interviewing some of the strangest people on the planet. I'd even had an alcoholic in full-blown DT's seizure on me one day. Big muscular guy. He hit the floor and I thought he was dead! That's when I learned to appreciate the real ER as the nurses and doctor jumped into action and had him on a table and medicated before I could wipe the horrified look off my face.

More than anything, I was going to miss the renewed sense of hope stirring in my gut again. Maggie and John had somehow touched me, rekindling my faith and genuine compassion for those less fortunate. Without a weekly dose of troubled souls to feed my spiritual rebirth, I wondered where my path would take me.

As I walked out of Faith General's back door, my father flashed before my eyes. Something he'd said to me when my college baseball days ended and I was confronted with the age-old question: what am I going to be now that I have to grow up? It might have been the greatest thing he ever said to me. "When one door closes, another one opens if… you listen with your heart."

I turned and took one last look back, then sped away, just as I'd willingly done twelve hours earlier with John riding shotgun. I had no idea where I was going. No idea how I'd pay my bills in six weeks if I didn't find another job. No idea what I was going to do, and yet…

I felt a strange peace overwhelm me. My heart was talking to me. Again.

This time I planned on listening.

chapter twenty-one

I PULLED INTO MY APARTMENT COMPLEX, overcome with fear, the thought of sitting home alone disgusting. My mind raced, my left brain demeaning me, forecasting my destiny — hawking homeless newspapers on the streets of Nashville. My right brain whispered, "Kick back,you reinvented yourself here in Music City. You can do it somewhere else." My heart challenged me to take a deep breath, close my eyes, *be still*, and know.

I turned around in the parking lot and puttered away, driving towards downtown. I cruised aimlessly, lost somewhere between the warmth of knowing that I could live with the choice I'd made to drive John home, and the stark reality that I'd just been fired in tough economic times because of it. I turned onto Lower Broadway, the honky-tonks having closed only a few hours earlier. I passed the mother church of country music — the Ryman Auditorium – I coasted a block down to the back door of Tootsies, where rebels the likes of Johnny Cash and Kris Kristofferson wrote and sang songs about losing jobs while downing a few cold ones.

I pulled over long enough to call my son, only to get the same answer I'd been getting for weeks — voice mail. I thought about driving to Knoxville but realized that I had no friends there anymore other than my mother and brothers. I watched the people hustling up Second Avenue, many in suits, apparently on their way to the capitol and the courthouse, or perhaps one of the many state office buildings or banks scattered about downtown. I sat in my car, realizing that outside of work, I had no real friends in Nashville. I had no one to turn to. And then it hit me again, a little harder than when delivered. I just got fired. Not downsized, or eased out the door. I was tossed out. Terminated, with absolutely no job prospects on the horizon.

I circled the downtown streets as real people with real jobs strutted to work. I passed by Printers Alley, wondering if one of the joints had an all-you-can-drink morning buffet. I crossed one of the Cumberland River bridges leading out of downtown and jumped back on the interstate. Fifteen minutes later, I found myself on familiar streets again, heading towards the only real friends that I had at the moment.

"I'm so sorry Michael," Maggie said, "I had no idea we'd cause you such grief." Her sad, tear-filled eyes told the story. "How can we help? I'll call the hospital administrator and... "

"It's okay," I comforted, lost in the irony of the moment – Fired for aiding and abetting her husband, and I'm here consoling. I figured they'd hear about my firing, and I wanted to make sure they heard it first from me.

I had another reason for driving out to see them. I knew Baxter would do whatever it took to get John back on the unit. I still didn't know why he wanted or needed him so badly. It didn't make sense that one patient could be that important to his research. But there was no doubt he wanted me out and wanted John back. What I had to do was prepare John and Maggie for what, in all likelihood, was going to happen. Baxter would demand that John be picked up by the police and brought back to the geriatric psychiatric unit. From a legal point of view, given that John was an involuntary patient at the time of his escape, Baxter and the hospital had every right to request that the police or sheriff's department intervene.

As tough as it would be for John and Maggie to endure another police ride down to the Faith General ER, I sensed the opportunity for a silver lining, a homecoming thirty years in the making, if I could persuade Jenny and Maggie to join me in the undertaking.

I sat on the back deck with John and Maggie, sipping coffee and basking in the warm sunshine as a solitary dove sang his lonely tune. As easy as it would be to mope about losing my job, I knew the time had come to take action.

I thanked Maggie one last time for preparing my treat — French toast, just like Mom used to make — and headed home. I smiled as their house disappeared in the rear view mirror, flashes of Mom and Pop before he passed and how they enjoyed taking rides together out in the country.

As I entered the main highway, warm memories of Mom stirred within, of our weekly grocery-shopping trips to the White Stores and lunch at the Krystal where we ate our miniature ten-cent burgers and fries out of boxes delivered on a tray that attached to Mom's side of the car.

I pulled up in front of my apartment wishing I had some place to hide other than home alone. My only salvation was the sheer exhaustion that suddenly smothered me. I unlocked the door, hurled my backpack on the kitchen table, curled up in a ball on my couch and passed out.

My phone awoke me from a deep sleep; my head pounding violently again. "Hello." I glanced at the clock. It was two-thirty in the afternoon.

"Michael." Maggie's voice sounded shaky. "They're here."

I sat straight up. "Just stay calm and remind John to go willingly," I assured her. "The police are not the enemy, okay? They're simply doing what the law dictates. Be nice to them, and tell John to do the same. We don't want to give Baxter anything to use against us."

"Do you think he'll have to stay long?" Maggie asked.

"His court date was set before he eloped," I said. "Tell John again to refuse to sign a voluntary consent for treatment. That way the court has to hear his case in four working days. They'll be no reason for them to get another date. They'll stick with the one they got."

"And after that," Maggie hesitated, still unsure of what the process entailed.

"It will be in the hands of the judge."

"They knocking," Maggie said, sounding frightened.

"It'll be okay," I reassured her. "Just get John through it without incident. How's he doing?"

"He had a restless nap after you left and seemed to forget where he was when he woke up. I coaxed him outside and that perked him up. I just hope he can hold up through all of this. His memory is not good, and he gets frustrated. I hope they don't try to upset him in court."

"He'll be fine," I assured her. "Just keep reminding him of what he has to do."

"Oh, I hope this works," Maggie said. "John will be so surprised."

"I'll let you know," I said and hung up. I took a deep breath and dialed the California number. "Let the games begin." I mumbled as I tapped my pen nervously on the coffee table, trying to convince myself that I could pull this off. The official term for the games: a probable cause hearing in Davidson County's General Sessions Court. On one side: Faith General Hospital. On the other side — John Robert Dalton, the patient. The issue: his competency and whether or not he should remain in the hospital against his will. The verdict: solely on one Davidson County judge.

That's how most probable cause hearings played out, what few there were to begin with. The vast majority of adult psychiatric patients admitted against their will signed a voluntary consent for treatment before the 96-hour deadline / court date came around. Those few cases that wound up downtown were almost always no-brainers — acutely psychotic or demented patients incapable of signing a voluntary consent, much less maintaining some sense of sanity outside the hospital. In those cases, the judge would grant the hospital an additional fifteen days of inpatient hospitalization to stabilize the patient. If, after fifteen days, the patient remained a danger to himself or someone else, then another hearing would be held.

Both sides had legal representation. The hospital sent their finest. The patient customarily had the court appointed variety. Both sides had ample time to present their respective cases, although ninety-nine percent of the time, the attending psychiatrist's recommendation was what the judge adhered to. He might ask the patient for his thoughts on the matter, but in most cases it was over in fifteen minutes, and the patient was carted back to the Faith General Hilton for another fifteen days behind locked doors. In theory, the system protected anyone, patient or not, from being locked away for an extended period of time in a mental institute or hospital without legal recourse. In reality, rarely would a judge rule against the hospital psychiatrist.

"Hello."

I froze at the sound of the soothing male voice on the other end of the phone line. My pulse quickened, my throat suddenly dried. I hadn't even rehearsed in my head what to say.

"Hello," the voice called out again.

"Yes... uh... is Matthew Dalton available?"

chapter twenty-two

I WASN'T SURE WHAT TO EXPECT as I pulled into the downtown Hilton parking lot. Talking to John's attorney via phone was tough enough. The thought of sitting across the table from him sent butterflies flitting about my insides. And it wasn't the case material that was spooking me. It was the role that I had assumed as peacemaker between John and his son, Matthew, the very attorney I was about to meet. I garnered that role the minute I phoned his San Francisco home and told him that his father needed him.

I stepped into the lobby and quickly located the elevators. It was time for me to go to work. I checked my files as I ascended to Matthew's room, making sure one last time that I had my case outline in the front folder. John's case was my lead into convincing Matthew to make amends with his father after thirty-three chilly years "Showtime," I whispered my work mantra as I knocked on the door.

"Michael?" he said, he being of obvious health and vigor, his solid six-foot frame and intense blue eyes a replica of his old man's stature.

"Yes." I extended my hand, momentarily stunned, wondering if my salt-and-pepper hair had the same manly hue as his. "I'm sorry." I shook his hand. "As much as I've heard about you, I've never seen a picture… " I looked down briefly, nervous, bordering on anxious, confused as to why I'd blurted out, but now that I had, I needed to say something.

"Looking more like the old man now am I?" Matthew said, graciously ushering me in and over to a small table in his suite. "You want a cup of coffee, or water?" he asked.

"Coffee's fine," I said as I set my files down in front of me. "Actually, seeing you for the first time sent flashes of what John must have looked like as a young man, and how he was quite the catch, as Maggie likes to say."

He sat across from me, a smile on his face. "I guess it is true, to some extent anyway."

"What's that?" I asked, relieved that he was smiling.

"How our generation swore that we'd never become our parents, or father in my case." Matthew sipped his coffee and looked up at me. "Is that a sign of wisdom? When we come to the realization that our parents weren't so bad and doing the best that they could do at that moment in time."

I felt the tension in my shoulders subside as I took a long deep breath.

"You okay?" he asked.

I looked at him and smiled. "I'm fine. One of the lucky ones," I said, raising my mug to him. "Very blest when it comes to parents."

We dove into John's case, and it didn't take long to realize that Matthew had done his homework in regards to mental health proceedings in the state of Tennessee. Within two hours, we were done.

Matthew turned towards me. "Is there anything else that we need to discuss between now and tomorrow morning?"

"No… well, yes," I stammered, clasping my files.

He shut his briefcase. "Please tell me the good-ole-boy legal system has nothing to do with what you're about to tell me."

"Actually, no," I said, baiting him as much as one can bait a veteran attorney who has made a career of fighting governments and corporations. "Well, sort of… "

He stood. "Okay."

"I did a little digging on the judge who routinely hears these cases," I said. "The Honorable Jimmy Jackson."

"With a name like that, I'm afraid to ask," Matthew mused.

"A descendant of President Andrew Jackson, no doubt," I said with a sly grin. "And apparently as shrewd and every bit as tough as his ancestry."

"You got my attention," Matthew said, "Have you had lunch?"

"Starving," I replied. "What are you hungry for?"

We sat outside at Centennial Park, feasting on deli sandwiches in the large field at the foot of the Parthenon, Nashville's full-sized replica of the Athenian temple.

"So tell me about this judge," Matthew said.

"It was attorney Jimmy Jackson's defining moment as a country-boy-turned big-time lawyer," I said, reaching for my Pepsi. "He defended a well-known moon-shiner in a Nashville murder case involving a wealthy socialite." I stopped and turned to watch, as did Matthew, as a pair of long-legged Vanderbilt coeds jogged by. "Oh, to be young again," I said, turning back.

"I wouldn't say no to a vacation back in time," Matthew said, a soft smile on his athletic face, perhaps reliving a Berkley moment on the heels of the sixties, quite the adventure for a twenty-two-year-old lad from the outskirts of Nashville.

I sat in silence with him, drifting back to my campus days at home in Knoxville, the fall leaves and football, the dogwoods in spring and baseball, and coeds of every size, shape, and color, including the post-Hippie gals who gravitated towards working with troubled kids.

"So your judge took on the high society crowd," Matthew said, "and what, won his case?"

"From what I've read," I said, "he embarrassed them with his knowledge of the law and his wit. That case spearheaded his career." I glanced towards the open fields of the park filled with walkers, joggers, workers on lunch break, and students tossing Frisbees and kicking soccer balls. "His dying commitment to the law earned the respect of the people and the wrath of those with money and power."

Matthew crunched on a baked potato chip, holding my gaze with fierceness in his eyes remnant of his mom's intensity. "How does that play into your notion of a death on the geriatric unit and not trusting the research?"

I wiped my mouth and reached for another swig of Pepsi. "Legend has it that a Music City money monger tried to put the old judge out to pasture on more than one occasion, but, he refused to retire or relinquish power to anyone other than the law itself."

"And his interpretation of it," Matthew said.

"Yeah, well, that's exactly what came into question several years ago."

"Meaning?" he asked.

I went on to explain how a local news investigative report claimed that an attorney in a prestigious law firm attempted to have Judge Jackson removed from the bench, citing the judge's dementia as detrimental to his ability to make sound legal decisions.

"And?" Matthew asked, stuffing the last bite of his sandwich in his mouth.

"The law firm had ties to a major healthcare corporation

based in Nashville," I said, "one that wound up on the wrong side of Judge Jackson."

"How so?"

"It was a personal damage suit," I said. "Judge Jackson ruled in favor of the individual and blasted the healthcare corporation for its blatant mishandling of the situation." I crumpled my sandwich wrapper and chips bag, stuffing them in a nearby garbage can. "The story branded our judge as a champion of the little man and one who did not take too kindly to corporations running roughshod over consumers."

We walked back towards my car. "I can paint my father as the little man," Matthew said, "caught in the crossfire of a renegade psychiatrist and a hospital desperate for research dollars. But..."

I opened my car door and slid in.

He joined me in the front seat. "Judge Jimmy Jackson is far too shrewd to be persuaded by anything other than the facts of our case, which I feel are solid in our favor."

I started the car. "As long as your father wakes up on the right side of reality in the morning." I cruised around the Parthenon, unsure whether or not to drive towards the hospital, or take Matthew back to his hotel room.

"You did say that the delusional episodes only occur as he's waking up from his afternoon nap, correct?" Matthew asked.

I nodded. "From what your mom's told me," I replied. "I just hope..."

"Me too," Matthew said. "Me too."

I killed about as much time as I could driving around the Vanderbilt campus, Matthew seemingly content to stare out his passenger side window at the west Nashville scene. I sat at a red light, yearning to talk about John. Matthew must have been on the same wave length.

"Does my father even know that I'm here?" he asked.

"I haven't told him," I said as I turned onto West End, heading away from his hotel room.

"How do you think he will respond to me?"

I glanced his way and smiled. "I think that has a lot to do with how you respond to him." I refocused on the road, glad that the downtown traffic was heavy and moving slowly. "I know your father reminds me of my dad."

"How's that?" he asked, turning in his seat towards me.

"Underneath that gruff exterior is a kind and gentle old soul." I stopped at another red light, touched by the memory of Pop. I looked straight ahead. "I recall my father not making it through a Thanksgiving Prayer at the dinner table when I was about ten years old."

"What happened?" he asked.

"He was giving thanks for our family and started crying." I cruised onward towards the Cumberland River bridges leading away from downtown, my eyes locked on the road, my mind replaying that scene thirty-something years ago. My father, the stern, no-nonsense, self-educated man who never laid a hand on me, yet, who I feared terribly, not for any threat, but out of respect and not wanting to let him down or anger him. There he was breaking down in front of Mom and his boys, their boys, my brothers seven and nine years older than me. I saw him crying and felt a sense of relief that he was, in some way, human too, with emotions and feelings. Over time, as my brothers followed their respective paths, including stints in the Air Force for both, just like Pop, I stumbled through adolescence, no longer fearful of challenging him on the social hotspots of the times – long hair, facial hair ala Joe Namath's Fu Manchu, the Viet Nam War, discrimination. As we both aged, our battles became more civil, and I saw my father as a veteran of World War II, a proud yet fiercely humble and private man, who honored God and family, and who mellowed dramatically over time in his perception of war and race and not judging a man by his looks.

We stopped at a red light in front of the refurbished Davidson County Courthouse, the bridge in sight. I delayed a bit when the light turned green, waiting to see if Matthew would redirect me. He did not. I started across the bridge.

"It's funny…" Matthew said as he glanced out his window at the river below. "Hey, who's the big white guy there?" He pointed to the giant poster-like picture hanging on the outside of the Tennessee Titans football stadium.

"Frank Wycheck," I replied, "a great tight end. He played in the Titans heyday back in the nineties with Steve McNair and Eddie George."

Matthew smiled. "He loved that team and their toughness."

"Who?"

"My dad," he replied with a sly smile.

"How'd you know that?" I fired back.

He turned my way. "Hey, I may not have spoken to the man in thirty-three years, but it doesn't mean I didn't ask about him." He smiled again, and then took a deep breath, as if letting out all the air he could muster.

"Maggie, ah, I mean your mom?" I asked.

"Who else." He took another deep breath, glancing around at his surroundings as I drove towards north Nashville.

"So what actually happened between you and your father?" I asked.

"He never told you?"

"Both he and your mom mentioned a falling out," I said, "but otherwise, no."

Matthew checked his watch. "It was a series of events, but it all started with me refusing to accept a scholarship to West Point."

"Oh boy," I said, glancing his way.

"Yes, indeed," he said with a sigh, "if you've spent any time with my father, you know how much God and country and defending her honor means to him." Matthew took a long look out his window before continuing. "It was a nasty argument. I said some things about the military and how Viet Nam was a prime example of this country's willingness to murder innocent people."

"I'm sure that went over well."

"My poor mother," Matthew mused. "She tried so hard to pull us together."

"So how'd you wind up in California?"

"Dad finally told me that if I refused to go to West Point on a free ride, then I could pay for my own college. Of course, I had to one-up his threat."

"What'd you say to him?"

Matthew snickered. "I said that I had no intentions of going to college. I was going to travel out west and see this country first." He laughed again. "I had to throw in a dig when he asked me what I would do if drafted by the Army."

"Ah yes, the old conscientious objector trump card, huh?" I said.

"Who told you that?"

I glanced his way and smiled. "Jenny."

He shook his head. "I should have known."

"So you didn't run off to Canada?"

"No," he emphatically replied. "Me and a buddy headed out west a week after high school graduation. My friend eventually came back as planned, but I stayed and fell right into step with the Berkeley scene, attended Cal-Berkeley and landed a part-time job in a law office run by a bunch of Hippies." He smiled, a look of joyful contemplation on his face. "The rest is history."

"And you never spoke to him again?"

"Not a word for the first couple of years, even though I

called Mom every week." He turned and looked out the window. "It hurt her so much, and I regretted knowing that, especially when he refused to come out to my wedding. After that, it was easier to talk to Mom and relay messages or holiday greetings to him through her."

"I can't imagine what she's feeling now, after thirty-three years."

"She's excited," Matthew said, "no doubt about that."

"And you?" I asked.

He shrugged. "Nervous, scared, wanting to make amends."

We drove in silence for a few minutes, Matthew seemingly lost in his family dynamic, me drowning in mine, wishing I could go back and spend more quality time with my father, wondering why, after feeling the loss and hurt that I felt when Pop died, that I had replicated with my own son such an aloof attitude about our relationship, or growing lack of one.

Matthew broke the silence. "So you really sacrificed your job for my father?"

"It was a no-brainer," I said.

"How so?"

"The look on his face when I found him hunkered down by my car," I said. "And then seeing his face, and your mom's, when I pulled into their driveway that night. Maybe they hit too close to home." I glanced over my left shoulder and switched lanes. "Your parents struck a nerve with me I guess." I slowed at the approaching intersection. "I just knew in my heart that it was the right thing to do."

"I'm glad they wound up with you," he said. "Mom and Jenny haven't stopped talking about what you did."

"Jenny?"

"She claimed that you were their guardian angel."

"She did?" I blurted out.

"That's not all she told me," he said, a big grin on his face. "So how'd you like it?"

"What?" I played dumb, although I wasn't sure what he was referring to and not real sure I wanted to go there.

"The tree house," he said, "our old fortress." Matthew leaned back, a joyful look on his face. "Sis and I had so many good times up there."

I drove onward, clutching the steering wheel with both hands.

"She told me about taking you out there in the dead of night," he said. "She said that you had never seen the woods like that before."

"It was eerie and beautiful at the same time," I said, staring at the road, unable to glance his way but wily enough to cover my anxiety. "One of those special moments that I'll remember the rest of my life."

"You didn't take advantage of my sister up there, did you?" he sternly asked.

"No." I shook my head, unsure if he was playing or serious.

He laughed. "Just kidding."

I glanced his way and smiled.

"Jenny thinks the world of you and what you've done for our parents."

"Feeling's mutual," I said, letting go of my death grip on the steering wheel.

"You wouldn't be driving me to the hospital by chance?" he asked.

"Actually, yes, I was." I slowed to stop at a red light. "But I can turn around… "

"No," he said, "it's time."

"You sure?"

Matthew nodded. "It's funny how things work out."

"What do you mean?" I asked as the light turned green.

"I've thought about this moment for the past ten years," he said, "but never could find a strong enough reason." He sighed. "When Mom called the night Dad was re-hospitalized, I knew that I had to come home. Somehow, some way." He leaned in towards me. "I just wasn't sure how it was going to play out, until you called. It was like a prayer answered, my friend."

I nodded and smiled, warmth enveloping me as we turned onto the two-lane road that led to the hospital. "You ready for this?" I asked.

Matthew turned towards his window, a slight quiver in his voice. "I think so."

chapter twenty-three

I DROVE PAST THE OLD HOSPITAL entrance, which had been blocked off years ago, and turned left at the next side road, only to turn into an alley and come back out onto what was once the grand entrance to Faith General's pristine grounds. I slowed, Matthew turning, as did I, to the left to see my favorite hiding-spot pond. I rolled my window down and eased across the road to get a closer view of the small family of ducks who hung out at the water's edge.

"There they are!" I pointed with little boy excitement to my two favorite ducks.

"Is that...?" Matthew smiled. "What is that?"

I laughed, my first hearty one in a long time, or so it seemed. "Afro Ducks," I said. "There's the one with a white Afro." I pointed. "See it?"

Matthew appeared to be enjoying the moment as well, his face inquisitive, like a little boy. He pointed. "His partner has a black Afro on a white head." He turned back towards me. "Are they some type of special breed?"

"I have no idea," I said, nodding to my web-footed friends. "Just two old ducks enjoying life together." I turned my gaze across the pond towards three weeping willows, their branches tickling the pond within earshot of a family of turtles sunning on their private floating log. My thoughts drifted back to one of my last walks around the pond — I was with Carol and feeling like a bumbling love-struck teenager, her touch and sultry smile electrifying my body; and yet, her presence on that day made me feel like I was walking with an old friend.

Matthew's voice brought me back to reality. "Is this part of the hospital's property?"

"Yeah," I said, "I try to sneak down here whenever I can."

"Did you ever bring my dad out here?"

"Sure did," I said as I watched a pair of squirrels scampering under two mammoth oak trees at the base of the bank leading up to a large, white-brick church, its stark-white steeple overlooking the hospital valley below and what used to be an innovative turn-of-the-twentieth-century sanatorium, complete with apple orchards and farmland to support its operation. "There was one day…" I smiled as I recalled my panic that morning, thinking the deceased patient on the unit might be John. "I found him down here."

"Did he escape more than once?" Matthew asked.

"No," I laughed. "Once was enough."

I eased back out onto the road, my mind drifting back to John's stay on the geri-psych unit, including meeting the cast of characters. "The church lady," I mused.

"The what?" Matthew asked.

"A diminutive lady up on the unit. We christened her the church lady," I said. "She was quite preacher, fire and brimstone included if she liked you."

Matthew looked at me puzzled. I quickly told him the story of the church lady and that eerie smile as she told me where to find his father. "Your father loved it out here," I said, "but couldn't wait to get home to your mom's rose garden and his beloved perch on the back deck."

173

I pulled into the back parking lot, caught somewhere between sweet memories and the sadness that still engulfed me about losing my job. I needed the money to survive, no doubt. Still, it was the patients that I was going to miss, and Carol, and my comrades as we faced the challenge of a twelve-hour-shift locked away in a standing-room-only fortress with deeply disturbed men, women, children and their families. As we approached the time clock entrance, I reached into my wallet and pulled out my ID badge.

"I thought they fired you," Matthew said, glancing around to see if anyone was watching us.

"They did," I said. "They're withholding my last check, a whopping one hour the day they fired me." I held the door open and ushered him in, dazed look and all. "I told them I'd be in soon to settle up."

"Why not just walk in the main entrance?" he asked.

"I was hoping I might see an old comrade back here," I said, motioning down the hallway to my right. I gazed at the psych admissions side door, wondering if they had hired someone to take my place, perhaps even someone attracted to Carol, or vice versa. The housekeeping office door down the left side of the hallway opened, momentarily startling me.

"Well, I'll be," a smiling face beamed. "They come to their senses and hire you back?" asked Juanita, a veteran housekeeper well-versed in the nitty-gritty dealings of Faith General's finest, both on-the-clock and beyond the parking lot.

"We're on a secret mission," I said with a wink. "You got my back?"

"I didn't see a thing," she said. "You take care of yourself, Michael."

"You too, Juanita," I said as I led Matthew down the back hallway.

We entered through the last locked door and hustled over to

the stairwell. Matthew scampered up the steps and stood waiting on me at the entrance to the second floor hallway.

Matthew gently grabbed my arm. "Are we in trouble if you are seen here?"

I slowly opened the hallway door. "Shouldn't be," I said as I locked my eyes on the geri-psych door entrance, the big red Elopement sign still hanging on the door. "Unless security or administration sees me."

We made it down the hallway without notice and ducked into the geri-psych family room just outside of the locked doors leading onto the unit. "When we go back out to the door, I'll hit the intercom and get the nurse on the line."

Matthew nodded, his demeanor suddenly distant.

"Just tell them you are John Dalton's attorney and the code number is twenty-four-twelve. You got it? Two four one two. I patted him on the shoulder. "You okay?"

He took a deep breath and smiled. "I wasn't expecting to be this anxious."

"It took a lot of courage for you to come this far," I said. "You won't regret having reached out to him."

He nodded. "Let's go meet my client."

I hit the intercom, Matthew eloquently spoke, code number included, and the door clicked open. "You ready?" I asked as I ushered him in.

The church lady pounced before the door closed behind us, blocking our entrance down the hallway, her eyes darting, her body stretching to meet Matthew's horrified face. "Repent you sinner!" She leaned her head back, never taking her eyes off of him. "For the end..." She raised her fist in defiance, prompting Matthew to step back against the wall. "It is near. It is now for you!" She howled in triumph and started down the hallway.

"Where's John?" I playfully called out to her.

She stopped and slowly turned my way, her eyes locked on

mine, a sly smile slowly forming on her withered face. "John the Baptist?" she asked.

"John married to Maggie," I replied, Matthew still frozen against the wall.

"Ah…" She cocked her head to one side, still holding my gaze, her grin widening. "The elusive one."

"Yes!" I said, edging closer to her, dying to hear her punch line.

She looked at me with that haunting grin. "He's gone," she whispered.

"Where?" I whispered back.

She pranced away, glancing back at me with those dancing eyes. "Gone to see Matthew!" she called out and cackled before disappearing down the long hallway.

I turned to Matthew, who remained glued to the wall. "You coming?"

He stood erect and nervously straightened his shirt, a dazed look still on his face. "How did she know my name?"

"There's no telling what that lady knows," I mused, cueing him to follow me down the hall. I checked the combination dayroom / dining room where John used to sit at the back table. There was no sign of him.

"Lord have mercy," a sweet and wonderfully familiar voice called out from the nursing station. It was Sally, my longtime favorite nurse on the unit. "Please tell me that they hired you back," she said in that rich, filled-with-love, Southern-black-woman voice that always brought a smile to my face. She stepped out into the hallway and gave me a hug.

"I wish," I said, "I truly do…" I introduced her to Matthew and asked about John's whereabouts.

"He's been in his room most of the day," she said, shooting me a look behind Matthew's back that warned me about John's condition. "He knows his court date is tomorrow," she said, "and seems worried about it."

"Do you have a room where we can talk with him?" Matthew asked.

Sally again glanced at me before answering him. "His roommate was discharged home this morning, so there's no one else in the room." She glanced down the hallway and then leaned into me. "I think Dr. Qualls is dictating in his office, and the social worker is interviewing somebody in her office."

"His room is okay." I nodded to Sally, not wanting to put her in a bad spot in case one of them, or perhaps even Baxter wandered onto the unit.

"Two-forty-five," Sally said, pointing down the hallway. "Next to the last on the right." She reached over and patted my shoulder. "Call me if you need anything."

"Thanks Ms. Sally," I said, "I appreciate it."

We started towards John's room, Matthew lingering behind me, taking deep breaths. I stopped right outside of the room and whispered to him. "Let me go in first and see how he's doing, okay?"

Matthew nodded.

"Look him in the eye and let him know that you love him," I said. "He'll respond." I took a deep breath, stepped into the doorway, and knocked loudly. "Hey there," I called out, glancing in at John lying on his bed, his eyes closed. "Anybody home?" I asked, waiting to enter out of respect and hoping that he recognized me.

I got no response.

I knocked louder. "John?"

"I heard you the first time," he growled as he slowly sat up and turned towards me. A big smile formed on his face. "Had you going for a minute, huh?"

"Don't do that to me," I playfully scolded as I shook his hand.

"You don't think I can handle this prison again?" he said, squeezing my hand.

"If you can deal with this place..."

"You got that right," he said. "I'm ready to go home."

"That's what we're here for," I said.

"We?" John stood next to his bed.

"I brought your attorney here to discuss the court hearing tomorrow. Is that okay?"

"Well, where is he?" He turned towards the doorway.

"He's..." I never finished, the look on John's startled face telling me what I needed to know.

"Hey Dad," Matthew said, standing tall and distinguished before his father. "Is it all right if I come in?"

I stepped back and watched as a proud old papa opened up his arms, and a fifty-five-year-old boy rushed to feel them wrap around his trembling body.

I stood with my head down, tears streaming down my face as father and son held one another, their thirty-three-year cold war fading away in the joyful sobs of two dear men.

John glanced my way and nodded ever so slightly, his watery eyes gleaming.

I smiled back at him and eased out the door, a soothing warmth in my heart, a yearning deep in my soul.

For my son.

chapter twenty-four

"ALL RISE," THE BAILIFF SAID. "In the mental health court of Davidson County…"

I glanced around the quaint courtroom, the tension for this proceeding far beyond that of the usual and customary hearings to determine the psychiatric fate of patients who remained involuntarily committed.

"Your Honor, these hearings are always closed to the public," pleaded Robert Willis, Faith General's young attorney. He was a northerner, fresh out of Vanderbilt Law, and Faith General was as good a place as any to ignite his corporate law career. He definitely looked the part in his slim-fitting jet-black suit.

"Mr. Willis, I'm well aware of the process," chided the judge. "Now, proceed." The Honorable Jimmy Jackson presided over his courtroom like a red-tailed hawk hovering over his prey.

"Your Honor, if the hearing is closed, then why are they here?" Willis gestured towards Maggie and me. We were seated at the long table next to John, who was proudly sitting next to Matthew.

"Mr. Willis," Judge Jackson slowly leaned forward, glaring over the reading glasses resting near the end of his nose, "if you'd bothered to check, you'd clearly know that Mrs. Dalton is the power of attorney for healthcare for Mr. Dalton." The good judge respectfully nodded his head at Maggie. "And Mr. Watson is Mr. Dalton's alternative healthcare agent, in case the Misses cannot fulfill her obligations."

"But..." Willis never had a chance to finish.

"Son, if you want to practice law in my courtroom, then I suggest you come prepared. The Tennessee General Assembly adopted the Durable Power of Attorney for Health Care Act years ago, providing both parties the right under the law to be present for this hearing, and that includes testifying if Mr. Dalton's attorney so chooses."

"Your Honor, I do have one concern before we proceed, if I may address the court," Matthew requested.

"This better be good," Judge Jackson said.

"Your Honor, we felt it vital to our case that Dr. Baxter be present since he was, in fact, the committing physician both times my client was involuntarily admitted to Faith General."

"So where is he?" the judge snapped.

"Your Honor," Willis jumped in, "Dr. Qualls has been the attending physician all along on this case, not Dr. Baxter. These hearings require that the attending physician testify, not the admitting physician. In most cases, the two are not the same, and there's no need to waste the court's time, much less the admitting physician's time, when the attending doctor is the one who is providing the treatment and best knows his patient."

"Proceed," Judge Jackson barked. "If, in the course of this hearing, I feel Dr. Baxter's testimony is crucial to my decision, then we'll cross that bridge at that time."

As was the norm, the attending physician was the first to testify. It only took ten minutes for Qualls to paint a picture of John as a good and decent man stricken with Alzheimer's, a disease that, if left untreated, could result in bodily harm and/or death to his wife or anyone present at the time of one of his delusional episodes. Led by attorney Willis, Qualls recounted John's attack on Maggie as well as his threats of physical harm towards the home health nurse and mobile crisis worker. He also cited a battery of harrowing statistics — cases where delusional spouses, left untreated, maimed loved ones. The focal point of their case — John's behavior stabilized when he was on his medication.

"One final question," Willis said, adjusting his tie. "Dr. Qualls, if Mr. Dalton were to successfully complete his treatment at Faith General Hospital, could his violent delusional episodes be treated such that he no longer poses the threat of bodily harm towards others?"

"If he continues with the course of treatment prescribed," Qualls said, "we could return him to his home and community and greatly minimize the risk of further incident."

"Thank-you Dr. Qualls. No further questions, your Honor."

"Counselor?" Judge Jackson gestured towards our table.

Matthew approached the witness stand. "Thank-you, your Honor. I'll be brief."

I glanced over at John and Maggie holding hands, their most significant unresolved issue standing before them, thirty-three years of yearning for this moment evidenced on Maggie's glowing face.

It had been a whirlwind thirty-six hours once Matthew arrived in town. I passed on Jenny and Maggie's invitation to eat dinner after yesterday's hospital visit that reunited the Dalton family. I had wanted to go, yet felt uncomfortable, as if imposing. I got the sense that Jenny was somewhat relieved that I declined their offer, perhaps uncomfortable with sharing her big brother since she rarely had the opportunity to spend time with him. Maggie actually seemed disappointed that I wasn't going to be there. A side of me did too, a deep-rooted sense growing within that the proverbial doors of opportunity my father spoke of were somehow connected to Maggie and John.

"Dr. Qualls," Matthew continued with his questions. "Are you saying that Mr. Dalton's medications are essential to his well-being and ability to live delusion-free?"

"Yes."

"What specific medication is he on for his condition?"

"Mr. Dalton is part of an experimental research..."

Matthew cut him off. "I'm well aware that he is involved in a research project run by Dr. Baxter. I'm also painfully aware that Dr. Baxter didn't want to face scrutiny about his project, so it leaves me no choice but to ask you questions about it. After all, you are simply carrying out his orders, correct?"

"Objection, your Honor, what is the relevance of such badgering?"

"Your Honor," Matthew ignored his counterpart, "I only have one more question for Dr. Qualls?"

"Can't wait to hear it," Judge Jackson mused.

"Dr. Qualls," Matthew turned his attention back to John's attending doctor, "what medications are you taking for your condition?"

"I beg your pardon," Qualls replied, white as a ghost.

Before Willis could spit out his objection, Judge Jackson motioned for both he and Matthew to approach the bench. "Son," he whispered, "I like your style, but I don't think this line of questioning is necessary."

"Your Honor," Matthew said, "I'm not trying to disrespect your courtroom or the doctor, but my client and his power of attorney for healthcare both question whether or not this physician is capable of judging the competency of another. We have reason to believe that Dr. Qualls is mentally ill with a diagnosis of bipolar disorder and suffers intermittent episodes of extreme mania coupled with delusions. If that can be established, then how can he be in a position to declare my client as incapable of returning home?"

"Tell you what gentlemen…" The good judge leaned back in his chair, dismissing the doctor from the stand. "Let's proceed with hearing what Mr. Dalton has to say and do so quickly. If I'm not satisfied, I'll ask him myself. And counsel," he looked at Matthew, "I don't need a parade of witnesses to determine if this man is able to go home."

"Yes sir, your Honor.

He looked at Willis. "Do you have any other witnesses?"

"No sir."

"Good!" He motioned to Matthew.

"Your Honor, I'd like for John Robert Dalton to take the stand."

Matthew gingerly walked his father through a series of questions to establish that he was alert and oriented and understanding what was being asked of him. John responded well to every question, looking at Maggie as he spoke each time.

In his cross-examination, Willis attempted to establish that John's delusional episodes had been under control while hospitalized and on medications.

"No further questions, your Honor," Willis said and returned to his seat.

Matthew stood. "Your Honor, may I ask my client another question regarding his medications?"

"Proceed."

Matthew quickly established the number of experimental pills John should have taken since his admission to the hospital and subsequent time at home. Since the medication was prescribed as once-a-day in both settings, it was easy to determine the exact number of pills that should have been missing from the bottle.

"Your Honor, I'd like for Dr. Qualls to take a look at this

prescription bottle to verify that his name is on it and the pills prescribed are, indeed, the ones in the bottle."

"This better be going somewhere fast," Judge Jackson said.

Dr. Qualls confirmed the prescription.

"Your Honor, if I may count the number of pills included here."

"The point, counselor."

"Your Honor, the point being that my client has never taken these pills. Not one! Not while he was on the unit and certainly not while at home. If you'd like to count these." Matthew turned towards Willis and Dr. Qualls. "What you'll find is that this 30-day supply, or thirty pills, issued at the hospital on the day he was discharged two weeks ago should have sixteen pills left if he'd been taking them at home as prescribed. Instead, what you'll find in that bottle is thirty-six pills. Thirty-six pills — six from his first admission on the unit and the thirty that were prescribed at discharge."

Matthew turned back to the judge. "Your Honor, my client never took the pills, not at home, not even in the hospital when the nurses were handing them to him every day. Not only that…" He turned and motioned to John, who pulled four more pills out of his pocket. Matthew strolled over and took the pills from his dad. "Here are the four pills from the past four days in the hospital," he said as he slowly dropped one pill at a time into the unused prescription bottle. He looked up at his father. "Can you tell us why you never took this medication?"

"I never trusted the doctor," John calmly replied.

"Dr. Qualls?" Matthew asked.

"No, he's all right, a little strange but okay. It was Baxter that I never trusted. I agreed to his research because I thought it would get me home faster. After that poor gentleman died, I knew that I'd done the right thing by not taking the pills."

Matthew smiled at his dad. "No further questions, your Honor."

"Counselor?" Judge Jackson barked.

"No further questions," Willis replied.

The judge stood. "Let's take a ten minute recess, and I'll render my decision." With that the Honorable Jimmy Jackson disappeared behind closed doors.

"Is he going to let my John come home?" Maggie whispered to me.

"I'd be shocked if he didn't," I replied.

"What makes you so sure?" asked Maggie.

"Your son."

"Matthew?"

"What a combination," I said.

"What do you mean?"

"Take the best of you and John, all the courage with class, the dignity with downright doggedness to do the right thing. Maggie, you should be very proud of your kids."

"I've been blest, Michael," she said, holding her gaze on me, "and so have you."

As the Dalton gang gathered around, anxiously awaiting Judge Jackson's return, I slipped out the courtroom door, eerily aware that in fifteen or so minutes, my life, or what was left of it, would return to normal, whatever that meant.

chapter twenty-five

TRUE TO HIS WORD, THE judge returned in ten minutes.
True to his legend, the Honorable Jimmy Jackson minced
no words. "Mr. Dalton, Ma'am." He nodded to them. "This
hearing was to determine whether or not you, Mr. Dalton,
continued to meet the involuntary criteria required to hold you
in the hospital against your will. Such criterion is solely based
upon whether or not you present a danger to yourself or others,
or if you are mentally or emotionally impaired to the point that
you have lost touch with reality and cannot care for yourself."
He looked right at John. "Mr. Dalton, I must admit that your
case concerns me. Based on your testimony today, you do not
meet the involuntary criteria to send you back to the hospital
against your will." He slowly leaned back, holding his gaze on
John. "I'm sending you home right now, but…" He turned his
attention towards Maggie. "It concerns me that you've taken
matters into your own hands and chosen to ignore your doctors'
orders regarding your medications."

John nodded. "I understand."

Judge Jackson continued. "I would highly recommend that
you find a psychiatrist or doctor, one not connected with Faith
General, and get another opinion on your condition. Do you
understand?"

"Yes," Maggie spontaneously replied for John. "We'll do just that, your Honor. We'll find another doctor to check him out."

"And take his medicines if the doctor so prescribes?" the judge said.

"Yes sir," John replied.

The judge leaned forward, his elbows on his desk, his hands clutched together and resting on his chin. "The courts can't hold you against your will for something that might happen. However," he looked at Maggie, "it frightens me that you might not be so fortunate the next time if he has another psychotic break. Are you prepared?"

"Yes, your Honor," Maggie said, "I am."

"If another such episode, as you call them, occurs, and involves a deadly weapon, then the court will not be in a position to send him back home. Is that clear?"

"Yes, your Honor," Maggie replied as she squeezed John's hand. "I understand."

Judge Jackson lifted his reading glasses from his face and dropped them on his desk. "You should seriously consider having a home health nurse or someone in the home in the afternoons when he wakes up from his nap." He turned back towards the hospital's attorney. "I'm sure the social worker on your unit can assist with a list of contacts and agencies that provide such care."

"Yes, your Honor," attorney Willis replied. "I'll make sure that happens."

"This hearing is adjourned," Judge Jackson said and abruptly disappeared into his chamber.

John and Maggie stood in unison, both of them beaming, as Matthew and Jenny surrounded them in celebration. "Let's go home," Maggie said.

"Oh no," John said, "after all I've put you through, we need to celebrate!"

"What did you have in mind?" Jenny asked.

"Lunch at Maggie's favorite restaurant," John said as he wrapped his arm around her, smiling at me as I watched from a few feet away. "Michael's coming too!"

"Yeah, partner," Matthew reached out and pulled me into the Dalton circle. "You up for it?"

I followed the Dalton car as we drove the short distance to the Spaghetti Factory. The closer we got to the restaurant the more I wished I was driving the other way. Alone. Cell phone off, music blaring. Just me and my thoughts, like what am I going to do for income? I liked my job, especially the three day work week. Pay wasn't bad. No on-call. Benefit package. Been in it long enough to understand the challenge and flow of a psychiatric ER. "Yeah right," I sneered, "knew it so well I lost my job." I shook my head in disgust as I slowed to catch the light, separating myself from the Dalton caravan.

I sat at the red-light thinking how romantic and rebel-like it sounded that I risked and subsequently lost my job for the rights of a patient. But did I do it for the right reasons? The light turned green and I coasted down First Avenue along the riverfront, watching as a smattering of homeless people sat smoking on the benches. Was I destined to wind up on the streets? I've lived on a paycheck-to-paycheck mentality for so long. I slowed again, hoping to catch the red light on lower Broadway, wishing I had the nerve to gracefully decline their lunch invitation. Hadn't I done enough for that bunch?

I eased into the parking garage, glad that I had separated myself from the Dalton's, still contemplating a way to bolt, recalling the absolute freedom I felt when I left my hometown of Knoxville and moved to Nashville. Why not move further west? I had no real ties here. Why not San Antonio? Or Santa Fe? Why not just drive until I ran into the Pacific? I always wanted to see this great country and swore I'd do it by car before I got too old to remember where I was going, much less recall where I'd been.

I pulled the visor down and looked myself in the mirror. "Why'd you do it?" I asked the man staring back at me. I studied my brown eyes, once so big as a tot that my older brothers called me headlights. I caught a glimpse of my soul seeping through my aging headlights, my heart reminding me that the happiest I had been since my divorce was the past month, and it wasn't because of Carol, or Jenny for that matter. "Although..." I smiled, checking my front teeth for foreign entities, realizing that spending time with attractive, articulate, and free-spirited women sure beat tapping my TV buttons alone.

I got out of my car and walked to the garage elevator. I pushed the down button and stepped back to the overlook facing Second Avenue. It was there that I got my answer. I saw Jenny and Matthew walk into the Spaghetti Factory while John and Maggie stood outside on the sidewalk, apparently waiting for me. The elevator door opened and I started to step in, only to stop. I let it go and turned back towards them, my vantage point partially hidden by the branches of a tree. I watched them cuddle below. I smiled, touched by the tenderness playing out before me, and stepped into the returned elevator, at peace for the time being, knowing that I'd helped an elderly couple in dire need at a time when I could have blown them off.

I stepped out onto Second Avenue and waved at them standing directly across the street from me. Maggie and John waved back, genuine looks of joy on their faces. I crossed the street and into their waiting arms. Maggie pulled me in close, John huddling beside me. "You were a godsend," she whispered to me, "an answer to our prayers."

"And the Good Lord will see fit to open another door for you," John said, wrapping his arm around me. "You hang in there," he said as Maggie patted me on my shoulder. "Now I don't know about you," he released me and reached for Maggie's hand, "but I'm ready to eat." They headed for the restaurant entrance. "Our treat," he said, glancing back at me, "so I hope you're hungry."

"Famished," I replied.

I was honored to join them for a victory lunch, yet felt out of place as they joyously played, "remember when...?" Who could blame them? There were a lot of laughs and childhood memories to relive. The radiant look on Maggie's face seemed to indicate the long grind well worth it, and yet, the year-to-year yearning, all those Thanksgivings and Christmas morns standing alone in her kitchen, praying, hoping, even talking to Matthew as if he was standing right next to her. As happy and fulfilled as she was on this blessed day, Maggie looked weary, as if the lifting of years of frustration, anger, hurt, and guilt over Matthew's hiatus freed her to lay that burden down.

"Mom, you okay?" Jenny asked, touching her on the shoulder.

"I'm fine," Maggie replied, reaching for her daughter's hand. "Just a little tired, that's all."

She clutched Jenny's hand, the two of them sharing an extended look into each other's eyes.

I wondered what mother and daughter were saying in that most precious of private moments.

chapter twenty-six

S EQUESTERED IN MY APARTMENT, I succumbed to my customary course of action when my back was against the wall – Jack Daniels in one hand, TV buttons in the other, phone ignored, responding to pizza delivery only, I brooded. I was drained, drunk and despondent.

My latest catnap on the couch had evolved into a rather pleasant dream when the ringing of the phone sank my sailboat cruising in the Caribbean.

"Michael, you okay?" a familiar voice called out.

"Yeah, I'm fine." I slowly raised up. "Where'd Jimmy Buffet go?" I muttered, shaking the cobwebs from my inebriated head.

"What'd you say?"

"Nothing." I rubbed my pounding forehead.

"Got a proposition for you."

"That's a scary thought coming from a slick lawyer."

Matthew's voice was enticing. "You'll like this one."

"Let me guess — you liked my work so much that you're offering me a six-figure salary to move to San Francisco and work for you."

"You're definitely dreaming," he laughed. "I'm a poor man's

lawyer these days, but you're right about your work. It was first class."

"Appreciate that."

"I'm offering more of a compensation package for the work you did."

"You don't owe me a thing," I replied, surveying the half-eaten pizza on the coffee table turned dinner table.

"You've made a lasting impression on my folks," Matthew said, "and Jenny thinks the world of you too. I was kidding when I said compensation package because there's no way to repay you for what you've sacrificed."

"So what's up?"

"Mom tells me you've become a Joe DiMaggio fan. Said she told you all about my father's dream to go to Yankee Stadium."

"And?"

"Dad and I want you to go with us to the Big Apple to see the Yankees play."

"You're kidding?" I stood up, suddenly energized.

"We're flying out on Thursday morning," he said. "Staying two days and flying back on Saturday. That will leave me enough time to get back home to California on Sunday."

"What about Maggie?" I asked, pacing the living room sidelines now, fired up about a trip to the Bronx and the ghosts of Babe, Gerhig, the Mick, and, of course, the man — Joe DiMaggio.

"She's the one who insisted that you go in her place," replied Matthew. "Said you would appreciate it a lot more than she would. Pop's excited about you going too."

"He is?"

"He's looking forward to continuing the DiMaggio versus Mays debate with you."

"Is Maggie okay?" I asked. "She spoke of how she longed

to see John's face when he finally got to fulfill his childhood dream."

"She's fine," he replied, "just tired. She's spent so much time and energy taking care of Dad that she's neglected herself. Jenny is going to stay with her while we're gone. Mom's looking forward to having someone look after her for a few days."

"I don't know what to say," I lied, knowing exactly what I wanted to say.

"Say yes! The trip is on us. A road trip for the Dalton boys and their favorite gunslinger," Matthew laughed.

"I feel like I'm imposing," I said half-heartedly. On one hand, I did feel that way. The cold war between father and son had just ended. This was John's dream, not mine. Why not let him savor it with his son? On top of that, they were offering to pay for me. Lord knows I couldn't afford two nights in New York on my wallet. Yet, the other side of me was saying, 'Do it! You just lost your job for him.'

Matthew, like his old man, went straight to the heart of the matter. "I need your help with him," he said. "You know him at this stage of his life far better than I do. And honestly, he's more comfortable knowing that you'll be there too. He trusts you, Michael. That's all he has talked about — how you put your livelihood on the line for him. He'll never forget that."

"What time is our flight?"

chapter twenty-seven

L OSING MY JOB ALMOST SEEMED worth it, seeing the look on John's face as we waltzed into Yankee Stadium on a late spring night in the Bronx. I wondered what was flashing through his mind as he sat mesmerized like a child in a movie theater for the first time.

"Dad, you okay?" asked Matthew.

John nodded and smiled, a boyish look of amazement on his face.

It was the top of the fourth when the Boston Red Sox clean-up hitter sailed a line drive over the Yankee's centerfielder.

John looked at me. "DiMaggio'd had that in his back pocket," he said, "and the thing is — it should have been a spectacular catch, but he'd make it look easy. That's how great he was. He'd run down balls that nobody else could touch." He leaned back in his seat and gazed out towards centerfield. "A style and grace that the grand ol' game hasn't seen since."

"Now wait a minute," I begged to differ, "you still going to argue with me that DiMaggio was a better outfielder than Mays? Willie'd get to balls that should have been in the gap for extra bases and wait on them with that basket catch."

"Not Mays, not Mantle, none of 'em had the grace of Joe,"

John said. "None of 'em!" He put his arm around me and whispered. "Means the world to me that you came along. Maggie too. I'm one blest man to have a friend like you." He leaned back in his seat, as gratified a look as I've ever seen on a man's face.

Matthew held his jumbo bucket of popcorn out for his father. "You okay?"

"Couldn't be better son," he replied as he inhaled a handful of popcorn "Couldn't be better."

It was one of the finest moments in my life. Sitting with the Dalton boys in Yankee Stadium, score tied in the bottom of the eighth inning, the crowd into it, the smell of popcorn, that magical sound — the crack of a wooden bat — as the Yankee's lead-off hitter smacked a shot in the left field gap, sliding safely into second base with a double.

"Mays would have gone into second standing up," I teased John.

"Joe'd gone in standing up..." He hesitated, his face aglow. "With a triple."

The Bronx Bombers won, the ghosts of Yankee icons smiling down from above. A tingling inside told me Pop was smiling too, proud of his son for helping one good and decent old man fulfill a lifelong dream.

chapter twenty-eight

"M om, you okay in there?"
Maggie emerged from the bathroom looking pale.
"Yeah, honey, I'm fine."

Jenny took one look at her and knew something wasn't right. Twelve hours had passed since the boys' departure for the Big Apple. Since that time, Maggie had done little more than lay in bed, overcome with weariness and flu-like symptoms.

Jenny placed her hand on her mother's forehead. "You're burning up."

"I'll be all right." Maggie sighed. "Probably just a virus."

"We're going to your doctor in the morning if you're not any better."

"There's little the doctor can do that rest and hot tea won't do," said Maggie. "I'm just sorry for you that you're stuck here with me."

"When's the last time you saw him?"

"Who?" Maggie asked, annoyed, well aware of who Jenny was referring to.

"Your doctor?" Jenny replied, stroking her mother's arm.

Maggie eased back into bed, the thought of seeing her doctor a frightening one. She hadn't paid him a visit in thirty years and had no plans to see him tomorrow. She was just fine and didn't need a doctor. Besides, she didn't have time to be sick. She had John to take care of. She placed Jenny's hand on her fiery cheek. "I'm sure I'll feel better in the morning," she told her. "Just be sure and wake me when your daddy calls." She eased back down in her bed. "And please, no word of this to him or Matthew. You hear me? I don't want them worrying about me."

"It's a deal," Jenny said as she touched her mom's face, "if you'll agree to see your doctor in the morning."

"We'll see." Maggie forced a smile and then closed her weary eyes.

chapter twenty-nine

I STOOD IN THE DOORWAY OF our connecting rooms, listening to John and Matthew converse with their spouses via phone, each sharing with childlike excitement his version of Yankee Stadium earlier in the evening. For a fleeting moment, I longed to have someone to share the joy and wonder with as well.

"Maggie doing okay?" I asked John as he hung his phone up.

"She's latched on to a bug of sorts," he replied. "She didn't want to tell me she was sick, but I could tell. Just like her to try and fake me out so that I wouldn't worry."

"Is it the flu?"

"Sounds like it," John said. "She'll be okay. She's tough." He sat down on the edge of one of the double beds in the room. "She rarely gets sick. Jenny said she'd take care of her and not to worry."

"I'm going to call it a night," I said as Matthew concluded his phone conversation. "You guys wore me out today."

Matthew laughed, turning towards his father. "Dad wore us both out." He reached out and touched his shoulder. "I haven't walked that much in years."

"Better get ready," John said, "cause we're hitting the

pavement early tomorrow. I got places to go before we head back to the stadium."

I looked at Matthew. "Pretty sad, huh? A 76-year-old man walking us into oblivion." I winked at John. "Good night folks," I said as I closed the door on our first night in the big city. Or so I thought...

It was two in the morning when the ruckus woke me up. I sat up, bleary-eyed, wondering who'd been whacked in the room down the hall. As I climbed out of bed, the door connecting our two rooms exploded with a fierce pounding.

"Michael! Michael!"

It was Matthew.

I slung the door open. "What's wrong?" I asked, only to find John pacing back and forth in a frenzied stupor. "What's going on?" I stepped into the room and right by a stunned Matthew. "John, talk to me." I said, standing slightly in his path.

He looked right through me as he passed by, never breaking stride, that same glassy-eyed look I'd seen in the ER seclusion room when he took a swing at me.

I stepped back. "Matthew, talk to me."

Matthew's hand trembled. "I woke up and found him standing over me," he said, his voice shaky. "Told me if I didn't get out of his house, he'd kill me."

"Did he take a swing at you?"

"No." Matthew shook his head vigorously, as if questioning what had just happened. "I thought he was going to." He took a long deep breath and watched, the initial shock in his eyes fading to sadness as his father paced the length of the room, seemingly lost in his delusion.

I turned back towards Matthew, "Something, or someone's voice eventually brings him back to reality."

"I thought he was coming out of it," Matthew said, "but

then he started up again. And that glare. Like he's looking right through you. What's going on?"

"He's delusional," I said.

"Meaning?" Matthew asked, regaining his composure.

"In his mind, he's at home and thinks we're intruders."

"So he's hallucinating?" he asked, watching his father's every move.

"I don't really know if he's seeing things that aren't there or hearing voices," I replied. "As far as we know, the only time he's like this is when he wakes up, usually from his afternoon nap." I watched John for signs of slowing down. "Whatever happens in his brain, he thinks the people around him are intruders. It's always the same scenario. That's what happened to your mom."

"So what do we do?"

"Wait and see," I said. "As long as he's just pacing and talking to himself, let's leave him be. We can try to talk to him, but I sure wouldn't holler or touch him."

"This is what Mom has to live with?" Matthew asked, shaking his head. "Maybe he should have stayed in the hospital."

I sighed, turning slightly, watching John as covertly as possible. "It's hard to say."

"Why can't they find a medication to stop this from happening?"

"There are anti-psychotic meds," I said, "but the patient pays a price with the side effects. And still, there are no guarantees."

He looked at me and then back at his father. "So how do you live with the threat of something like this?"

"Ask your mom," I said. "She's been doing it for the past several months."

"That long?" Matthew blurted out. "I thought..." He stopped as John turned towards him.

"Hey John," I called out, "how'd you like that ballgame tonight?"

He looked at me, appearing puzzled, as if torn between two worlds.

I played my trump card. "Maggie sure enjoyed hearing about it from you."

John cocked his head, glancing at Matthew, then back at me. "What's going on?" he asked, rubbing his eyes.

Before he had a chance to get worked up again, I explained that he'd had a bad dream, woken up confused, and Matthew was concerned. I assured him that he was okay now, and we could all go back to sleep.

"What time is it?" John asked.

"Two fifteen, Dad."

"We're getting up at six," John snapped, his ornery self back in the same time zone.

"Maybe I'll just leave the door open," I said, nodding to Matthew as I started back to my room.

"You don't snore real loud do you?" John called out, already underneath the sheets.

"Like an old bear," I laughed. "Good-night you old geezers."

"Same to ya!" John fired back.

Minutes later, with John sound asleep, Matthew and I slipped out on the tiny deck for a breath of fresh air.

"How does Mom do it?" he asked.

"She told me that her faith was all she had to get her through some nights," I said. "But it goes beyond faith. That's love, as pure and unconditional as it gets."

"She made it sound like it was no big deal."

"That's what mothers do," I said. "Take the weight of the world on their shoulders so their kids don't have to worry or even know what's really going on."

"Can't they do something at the hospital?" Matthew asked.

"Short of filling him full of anti-psychotic meds...That's the irony of Baxter and other researchers."

"What do you mean?"

"On one hand, they're playing mad professor with humans as lab rats," I said. "Yet, without those early experimental trials, we'd never have the miracle drugs that we now take for granted." I looked out across the parking lot. "I hope and pray they find a cure or a vaccine for Alzheimer's, but until they do, there's no stopping it. It's a degenerative brain disease, and there's no going back."

"You think Dad…?" Matthew turned his gaze towards the barren parking lot.

"I don't know," I said, the cool air sending a shiver down my spine. "He has some of the early signs and symptoms, but he's also seventy-six years old. How do you tell the difference between old age and Alzheimer's until it's too late?"

Matthew gazed back at his father. "So what do you do?"

"I know your parents have promised each other to do whatever it takes to stay at home and not in some sordid nursing home."

"That sounds all well and good," Matthew turned back towards me, "but what happens if Mom can't take care of him? What happens then?"

"That's a question thousands of families confront every day." I leaned over the railing, spotting our rental vehicle just below us. "Everyone wants to die a peaceful death at home, but the cold, hard reality is that most die with strangers around."

"Strangers?" he asked.

"Three-fourths die in hospitals," I said, watching a stray cat peruse the parking lot below. "Most being treated by docs they don't even know."

"I hate to admit it…" Matthew leaned back and took a deep breath. "Unless Jenny's talked with them, I know nothing of their plans about what they want to do. Even though Dad and I weren't communicating, I called Mom every week. Jenny did too. Yet, my guess is she knows less about it than I do." He placed his elbows on the railing. "Why is that?" he asked me. "Why is it you know more about what my parents want than I do, and you've known them what — a month?"

"It's easier to talk to a stranger than your own kids about dying," I said. "My parents never told me a thing, and from what I've observed and read, that's usually the rule rather than the exception."

"So how do you talk...?" He turned back towards John. "Sleeping like what happened fifteen minutes ago..." He slowly shook his head. "How am I supposed to approach that proud ol' soldier and talk about his death?"

"I don't know," I said, touching his shoulder, "but you and Jenny need to and soon."

"Why's that?"

"You may not get another chance," I replied. "If your dad truly has Alzheimer's, then he will die from it unless a vaccine or some miracle drug is developed and soon. Even then, his memory will be one of the first things to go and that's already happening."

"You've seen evidence of it?"

"To some extent, but I think he's done a heckuva job hiding it from you and Jenny."

"Hiding it?"

"He's old school," I said. "Just like you said — a proud ol' soldier." I stepped back from him. "He and Maggie, my parents, that generation learned to keep their problems to themselves and get on with the business of surviving. They're not about to change now."

"I can relate," Matthew said, a reflective smile on his handsome face.

I looked out across the parking lot, the stray cat long gone. "I think that's why they asked me not to give up the role as the alternative power of attorney for healthcare," I said. "They know I'll fulfill their wishes and not put you or Jenny in a position to have to make a tough decision."

"Yeah, well…" He glanced back at the vacant lot. "I still have a hard time seeing Mom and Dad as invalids and incapable of taking care of themselves."

"Happens every minute of every day," I said. "And the nursing home circuit, unless you're wealthy, is not where you want your parents dying."

"Maybe when we get back Jenny and I can approach them," he said. "Would you be willing to help us out before I fly back to California?"

"Sure."

Matthew smiled. "That's the least you can do for this family," he said.

"Yeah," I laughed. "No need to check my calendar for appointments."

He patted me on the shoulder. "I'm sorry, and grateful for all you've done. I can see why Dad responds to you."

I shrugged. "I just did the right thing for the right reasons."

"Yeah, but how many others would lay it all on the line for a stranger?"

I shrugged again, smiling all the while, warmed by his compliments.

"So why'd you really do it?" Matthew teased. "Did you tweak their will, or transfer funds to some offshore account?"

"Me?" I cried. "I'm technologically challenged," I said as I grabbed the door handle. "I finally took my old man's advice and listened to my heart."

Matthew followed me back inside. "A man of principles, huh?"

I stood in the doorway separating our two rooms. "Your folks reawakened that childlike exuberance and joy for life that

I once knew." I stretched my aching back. "How many middle-aged men can say that and really mean it?"

"Most of the ones I know are filthy rich, married three times and hollow inside," he said.

"A feeling I know all too well," I said, "the emptiness inside, not the rich part."

Matthew eased over to where John continued to snooze away. He reached out to touch his shoulder but pulled back, apprehensive, yearning to make a connection with his father, yet fearful of waking him up in the moment. He slowly pulled away and turned towards me. "I'm glad my parents have had such a positive impact on your life," he said. "I hope your relationship with them continues."

chapter thirty

"YOU 'BOUT READY MOM?" JENNY called out.

Maggie took a deep breath. "I'll be out in a minute." It was the last thing she wanted to do. He was a nice man and a good doctor, but she, like John, didn't want to know too much. As long as she was getting around and doing the things she liked and needed to do, why worry with a doctor?

Maggie turned her bedroom light off and started for the living room, only to stop. She flipped the light back on, stepped over to her dresser, and reached for her favorite framed picture, tracing the outline of the three figures standing in that old tree house out back. "Oh John…" She smiled, admiring the childlike grin on the man she'd dedicated her life to, his arms draped around Matthew and Jenny, both beaming with joy. She gazed into each child's eyes, basking in the warmth of knowing all was well with her family. "Thank you." She glanced at the small wooden cross hanging just above her dresser.

"You coming?" Jenny called out from the kitchen.

"Be right there." Maggie set the picture back on its small stand, touching their faces one more time. "Love you." She flipped the light out again.

Jenny put her arm around Maggie as they approached the car. "You hate this don't you?"

"Yes, I do," she said, leaning into her daughter, the added support much needed, even though she would never admit to such. "I'm feeling better this morning," she said. "I really think it's okay if I don't go." She glanced up at her daughter and meekly smiled, the same expression that Jenny, as a young teen twenty years earlier, displayed when trying to manipulate her mom into getting her way.

Jenny pulled her mom in close. "I've already called Dr. Richards, and he wants to see you." She stroked her mom's head. "He said he hasn't seen you in years."

Maggie wiggled free and sighed, her head down, frustrated, yet knowing all too well that her daughter was looking out for her best interest. "I haven't been sick in years, and I'm not so sick that I need to go now."

"We're going and that's that," Jenny said, opening the passenger side door. "You don't want to be laid up in the bed when Daddy comes home do you?"

"No." Maggie forced a smile as Jenny secured the seatbelt for her.

chapter thirty-one

I AWOKE ON MY COUCH, JUST as I had done the past two mornings, or afternoons, depending upon how late I'd been out the night before. After four solid weeks of searching for a comparable mental health job, I was hitless, hopeless and hellbent on proving to the middle management supervisors hiding behind their cyber desks that I was worthy of being hired. I had joked about living from paycheck to paycheck in the past, but this was fast becoming no laughing matter. I was six weeks from homelessness and growing despondent, so much so that I told the admissions director at the state mental institute that I'd work weekends and nights. He looked at me like I was crazy, assuming, I guess, that I was either too slow to keep pace during the day hours, or too desperate for a job, which I was fast becoming.

I tossed my two-day-old jeans towards the ever-expanding heap of soiled clothes and stumbled into the bathroom. I stood motionless in the shower and let the hot water pound the back of my neck, relieved that my binge would not extend to a third night out tonight. I'd had enough of the honky-tonk scene and had no problem admitting to myself that my playing days were over. I raised my head, the warm water pounding my forehead, all too aware that there's nothing more disgusting than a middle-aged man hanging out in a young gun's bar.

I stepped out of the shower and glanced at the man looking back at me in the mirror, wondering if I had the intestinal fortitude to step up to the plate and get a hit. Otherwise, I ran the risk of becoming a bummed-out bitter recluse. I slid over to my nightstand and grabbed my wallet, counting what cash I had left. I stashed the money back in its place, slid my son's picture out into my hands, and studied his handsome face, wondering what I needed to do to reach him.

I got dressed and sat down at my desk amongst the various folders and job applications I'd printed out. Within minutes of perusing the internet for job opportunities, the temptation to take one more day off burned within. "And do what?" I chastised myself. "Wind up in some dive again? Is that what you're made of?" I slammed a folder down on the desk, walked over to the front door and stepped outside, the warmth of the sun trumping the familial and financial strife gnawing at me. I stepped back inside, grabbed my keys and eased back out the door, the urge to walk overwhelming. Within minutes, I was strolling along a quiet sidewalk, enmeshed in the silence of the moment as a cool breeze rustled the leaves.

I walked back to my apartment with a renewed sense of hope and sat down to start the job hunting process again. Twenty minutes later the phone rang.

It was Jenny. I slumped in my chair, taken back by the news. Apparently the Dalton boys and I returned from our Big Apple excursion with the Bronx Bombers to a bomb that exploded much closer to the Dalton home, the kind that rips lives apart and leaves loved ones scrambling to deal with the fallout.

Maggie's trip to the doctor, the trip that she didn't want to take, the one that she somehow knew not to take, triggered a battery of blood work, which triggered a battery of scans and screens and tests, which detonated the C-bomb — cancer, hepatocellular carcinoma, a rare form of liver disease. A disease known all too well in third world countries and not that uncommon in longtime alcoholics with cirrhosis, yet, still lethal in the civilized and sober world. It is rare in that those stricken have no apparent liver disorder and, in Maggie's case, no acute symptoms. By the time it is diagnosed, the damage has been done and little if anything can stop it.

"What's the prognosis?" I asked.

Not good," Jenny replied. "Six months tops."

She went on to tell me how Matthew and John were ready to escort her about the country looking for the latest cure, but Maggie would have no part of it. Two doctors telling her that she had six months to live was enough poking and prodding to satisfy her. Besides, she had John to take care of, and as long as he needed tending to, she'd do the best that she could do.

"How's John holding up?" I asked.

"He was in a state of shock," Jenny replied. "That lasted about a week. Since that time, he and Mom..."

"What is it?" I asked, hearing the pain in her voice.

"It's like the two of them rallied around each other and pushed me and Matthew away."

"Would you expect anything different from them?" I asked, stepping into the kitchen to pour a glass of sweet tea.

"What do you mean?" she asked, sounding hurt by my comment.

"Their love for you and Matthew," I gingerly replied as I returned to my desk. "The last thing they want to do is disrupt your lives, not to mention their grandkids."

There was silence on the other line.

I continued. "I can see Maggie shooing you out the door," I said. "They're proud folk, Jenny. They aren't about to lie down and have their kids fretting over their every move."

There was silence again.

"Jenny…"

"I'm here," she blurted out, sounding as if she was fighting to keep it together.

"You know your parents will come up with some type of game plan," I said.

"I know. Mom always finds a way."

"Did she know that you were calling me?"

"Oh yeah, and not real happy about it either."

"What'd she say?" I asked.

"To let you get on with your life," she said. "Speaking of which, any news about a job?"

"Still looking," I said. "I had no idea that I'd be viewed as over-the-hill and expendable."

"Maybe over-the-hill when it comes to tree climbing," she teased.

"Hey, wait a minute now," I said as I stepped back outside.

"That will always remain one sweet memory," she said.

"Me too," I said, enjoying, if only for a fleeting moment, the goose bumps exploding on my skin. "Hey, you tell Maggie I haven't had a home-cooked meal in four weeks and won't take no for an answer."

"She'll like that."

chapter thirty-two

WITH MOON ROOF OPEN AND music blaring, I leaned into the last few curves as the sun offered one final glimpse at a western sky spattered with pinks and purples, oranges and blues, the thinly layered clouds creating an ever-changing hue no photograph could recreate.

I pulled into the Dalton driveway, just as I had done on a number of occasions, although it had been nearly a month since I'd spoken with either one of them. I turned the engine off and sat in my car, a side of me yearning to hug their necks, another side of me hesitant, not sure how to react to the news about Maggie. This wasn't work related anymore. It never really was. Maggie had me the first time those hazel-colored eyes peered deep into my soul, the connection between Maggie and Mom powerful. And John was like Pop in so many ways.

I climbed out of my car and started for the front door, stopping in the yard to enjoy one last look as dusk slowly blackened the eastern sky. "Give me strength," I murmured to the heavens as I stepped up on their front porch.

The door slowly opened. We reached for the storm door at the same time, my heart fluttering. I opened my mouth but there were no words. I stepped into the foyer and into Maggie's arms, overcome with emotion, my tears flowing freely as she consoled me like I was her little boy.

"Sorry." I stepped back and pulled my faded handkerchief from my back pocket. "I wasn't expecting…"

"You're a special man, Michael," she said. "Don't ever forget that." She grabbed my arm. "You hear me?" She gazed into my eyes and smiled, patting my hand.

"Yes ma'am," I nodded, clearing my throat. "Now get me into the den before I start again."

She latched onto my arm and escorted me into the kitchen. "John has been so excited that you were coming."

"Me too," I said, glancing towards her stovetop. "That smells delicious." I stopped and savored the sights and aromas of a Southern-fried kitchen, complete with made-from-scratch cornbread in the oven and fried okra in the cast iron skillet.

"Hey young man!" John called out from the den.

"Hey old man!" I playfully replied, smiling at a beaming Maggie before stepping down to greet him.

He slowly stood from his lounge chair and reached for my hand. "Where have you been?" He squeezed hard, a man's handshake to say the least, his left hand grasping my shoulder.

"Tryin' to find a job."

"Sweet tea?" Maggie called out from the kitchen.

"Yes, please," I nodded as I sat down on the couch across from him.

"Tough out there right now isn't it?" he said.

"Worse than I thought," I said, "a lot worse."

"When's the last time you had a home-cooked meal?"

"The last time I was here," I said, reaching for my glass. "Thanks." I said to Maggie as she handed me a tall glass of perfectly brewed sweet tea, complete with a fresh slice of lemon attached to its rim.

"We're in for a special treat tonight," John said, reaching up to stroke Maggie's face as she set his glass on the end table next to his Lazy Boy. "Chicken and dumplings," he said, playfully shooing her back to the kitchen. "They put the Cracker Barrel's dumplings to shame," he said, loud enough for Maggie to hear and cast a sweet smile back his way.

"Now that's some serious dumplins," I said with a smile her way as well, the tension in my gut gone as I turned towards the baseball game on TV. "Who's playing?"

"Reds and Pirates, Reds down four to two," John said, "bottom of the fifth, two men out, bases full."

"Who's at the plate?" I asked.

"Jay Bruce."

"Never heard of him," I said.

"Tough kid," John said, as if providing a scouting report on the Cincinnati Reds strapping right fielder. "Plays hard, a thirty-plus homer, hundred-RBI man." He took a slow drink of his tea. "Has a tendency to strike out a lot."

"I don't know these players anymore," I said. "They switch teams so fast in search of the big contracts."

"Makes you sick, doesn't it?" John said. "Guys hitting two fifty with fifteen homers making five million a year?"

"That's crazy," I said, nodding my approval as the count went full to the batter.

"They'll be running," John said, easing up in his chair to watch the wind-up and the pitch. "C'mon..." He sighed and slumped back in his chair.

"At least he went down swinging," I said, referring to the batter striking out to kill the rally. "I can't stand to see these guys strike out with the bat on their shoulder."

John nodded and smiled, delighted with our conversation about the game we both cherished.

I leaned back, took another giant swig of Maggie's sweet tea, and raised my glass. "Just like Mom used to make," I said, memories of me and Pop watching Sunday afternoon games together while Mom prepared an after-church feast.

"That's good tea," John said, waving at Maggie in the kitchen. He leaned forward, cueing me to lean in. He whispered. "You'd never know…" He took a minute, his face quivering ever so slightly, as if fighting back tears. "She's amazing Michael. The toughest, most loving, humble and gracious woman and wife that any man could ever ask for." He leaned back and took a deep breath.

I wasn't sure what to say. Then again, it was peaceful to be in the company of a friend who didn't require any response from me.

An hour later, the three of us sipped coffee on their back deck, enjoying the occasional shooting star flaring across an unseasonably cool summer sky.

"Who's ready for dessert?" Maggie asked.

John and I followed Maggie into the kitchen like pampered, old, house dogs. We sat at the counter and devoured her banana pudding filled to the rim with vanilla wavers.

As we sipped one last shot of coffee, Maggie turned towards John, who subsequently turned towards me. "What happens if you don't find a job?" he asked.

"I don't know…" I hesitated, embarrassed to share with them the sad facts that I had no real savings account as back-up and barely enough money in my checking account to last two months.

"What is it?" John gently prodded.

His fatherly concern, coupled with Maggie's compassionate gaze, broke down any remaining reservations I held onto. As much as I tried to convince myself that I didn't need anyone, I longed for human contact and someone who cared for me.

"I'm worried," I blurted out, sharing without hesitation or remorse that for the first time in my working life, I feared for the future, at least here in Nashville, where tough economic times produced a flooded market of applicants for even entry level positions. "They don't even have the decency to say, 'You're over-qualified.' "

"What do they say?" Maggie asked.

"That's just it," I said as I took another sip of coffee. "They send form-like e-mails telling me how much they appreciated…" I set my cup down. "And, of course, with all sincerity, if any other jobs open up, they'll call me."

"And never even speak to you?" John asked.

"Welcome to the 21st century," I said with disdain. "There is no human factor in the hiring process anymore."

"What do you mean?" Maggie asked.

"They review applicants on line, and I'm guessing that when they see my age and years of experience…" I leaned back and hung my head.

"Well…" John put his hand on my shoulder and nodded to Maggie. "I guess this is as good a time as any to share an idea Maggie and I had involving you."

"Me?" I playfully threw my hands up in the air. "What? Are we going to become bank robbers? Steal from the rich and give to the poor, minus a nominal fee of course." I smiled at the two of them grinning back at me. "We've got to come up with a catchy name."

"What we have in mind," Maggie said, "is a little closer to home."

"Yeah," John said, "like our home."

"And?" I nervously asked.

"We'd like to offer you a full-time job," Maggie said.

I backed out of their driveway and headed home in the pitch-black of night, my mind reeling. On one hand, their job proposal came as a total shock. In exchange for a reasonable monthly salary, room and board, and all the food I could eat, I would move in as the primary caretaker for John and Maggie.

I laughed as I coasted through the blinking yellow light leading back to the highway. Their job offer really wasn't that far-fetched. It was hard to argue economically. If I didn't find a similar job, I'd be back to hustling multiple part-time jobs and paying a small fortune for Cobra benefits.

I eased the moon roof open, wondering if I could stomach multiple work sites and being perceived as nothing more than part-time help. If I returned to Knoxville, I could possibly move in with one of my brothers until I found work and got a place of my own. Then again, as much as I loved my brothers and vice versa, I wouldn't want to be on the other end of such a request. Why do it to them? Otherwise, short of heading west, which, even though I fantasized about it, frightened me to no end, I was destined for the Salvation Army and sleeping with some of the same down-and-out patients I had assessed over the past few years.

My mind raced again, picking apart all of the "what if…" scenarios their job offer ignited. What if I needed to take a break and take a long ride in the country? What if I wanted to go out? I'd ignored Carol's phone calls up to now, but I longed to see her and find out if our once-budding relationship had anything left. What if I could no longer handle Maggie's illness from a medical standpoint, much less John's? Who's to say he wouldn't wake up from one of his naps and come after me? And what if I finally found a job and they needed me to start immediately? What then?

I pulled into my apartment complex, wondering how much the landlord would charge for exiting a few months early on my lease. And what if I moved in with John and Maggie, and five months later, needed to find another place to live because Maggie had died and John could no longer be safely managed?

"And guess who gets to make that call?" I moaned, knowing that if I took their offer, John and Maggie wanted me to maintain my role as back-up power-of-attorney for healthcare, not just for John, but for Maggie too. How would Matthew and Jenny feel about that? I can't imagine an assessment specialist, in a psychiatric ER no doubt, winding up as my Mom's power of attorney for healthcare. No way.

"And yet?" My heart countered as I sat at my makeshift desk sipping coke, minus the Jack Daniels for a change. I leaned back in my rickety office chair and glanced at an old picture that I'd recently discovered on my last visit to the home I grew up in. Mom and I were alone that day, sitting at the miniscule dining room table browsing through old picture albums and reliving fond memories. The picture that Mom and I found that day was an old black-and-white shot of me at the age of two. I'm in my hitting stance, a slight crouch from the left side of the plate ala Pete Rose, my hands squeezing a small wooden bat, a made-to-size Louisville Slugger for the tiny tot that I was. I'm wearing baggy white underwear, no shirt, bee-bop-looking shoes with thin, white, pull-up socks, and the bill of my Sox baseball hat is snugly pulled down on my forehead. My face is slightly tucked and locked in, my intense eyes staring out just above my right elbow at what would be the pitcher, or in this case, Mom taking the picture, or so she told me with a gleam in her eye.

As I leaned in to get a closer look at the childhood picture of myself now taped to the outside left edge of my computer screen, my heart softened, my breathing slowed, my mind exhaled, and the reason for taping it up there came into focus — to challenge me to rekindle that childlike joy and inquisitive spirit for life. Warmth filled me as I gazed into my innocent yet intense and fearless eyes, ready for whatever pitch came my way.

I still had questions, doubts, and fears about taking on the responsibility of caring for them, one of which I had asked them pointblank. "What happens if Maggie dies?"

"We'll do the best we can with the time we have left together," they had countered, "and leave the rest in God's hands." They assured me they would be prepared and not leave me hanging if and when the time came that John needed to be moved out of the home. "Or," as John said, "you might decide to stay put here with me. You're welcome to stay."

chapter thirty-three

I ROAMED THE GROCERY STORE AISLES alone, enjoying the freedom to meander, provided I did not receive a #911 call from Maggie or John. I had moved in with them three weeks before and had quickly fallen into both daily as well as weekly routines, including today, Wednesday, double coupon day. Maggie insisted, in a nice way of course, that I utilize the coupons that she cut out of the Sunday paper. Who was I to disagree? I was shopping with house money, eating quite well under their roof, and learning to cook the way Mom used to cook, minus a tinge or two of salt and fatback.

On her good days, Maggie taught me to make and bake old time goodies like roast beef surrounded by succulent new potatoes, sweet corn, carrots and green beans, the meat so tender that I could cut it with a fork. And of course we added skillet-fried cornbread and topped that evening off with made-from-scratch lemon meringue pie. Oh, if Mom could see me now, dabbling and baking in a kitchen big enough to move about freely.

The rest of my structured work time at the Dalton compound fell right into place as well. Utilizing my old teacher-counselor skills, I drew each of them a wheel and started filling it in with spokes — community support systems specific to each one's needs.

Pretty soon, I had a host of volunteers, home health nurses, and church members from John and Maggie's longtime congregation coming in at scheduled times to assist or simply visit. I even had John and Maggie giving me ideas on what would make life easier for each of them. If possible and within our working budget, I'd make the necessary phone calls, complete whatever paperwork, and stay with it until we could draw another spoke in either John's or Maggie's support wheel.

Most nights, after supper and kitchen clean-up, I was basically free, except for assisting as needed and administering the evening meds, making sure John swallowed the chemical cocktail designed to squelch his delusional episodes. Most evenings up until about ten, John and I flipped back and forth between ball games while Maggie stretched out on the couch dosing in and out, seemingly more and more of late, her powerful medications zapping her energy.

If I wanted privacy, or felt like they needed it, I simply retreated to my bedroom where I had a laptop and a small TV. They were asleep most nights by ten, and I rarely went to bed before midnight, providing me ample time to surf the internet for jobs or even tiptoe back out to the kitchen and the main TV in the den where I feasted on whatever sweet goodies John and I hadn't devoured earlier.

Surprisingly, life was good. Simple. Purposeful. And I must say I didn't miss Jack Daniels one bit. Not that either would have minded me taking a nip. I just hadn't done it and hadn't realized how much I was doing it until I started waking up with a clear mind and a zest for whatever the day might throw my way.

With my buggy overflowing, I tootled towards the check-out line, eager, as always, to peruse the tabloids oozing with twisted love triangles and alien contacts. My eyes had moved on down the line to Penelope Cruz' striking face, not to mention her sumptuous low-cut dress that adorned the cover of the latest Cosmopolitan, when my phone vibrated in my pants' pocket, jolting me back to reality. I pulled and finally yanked it out of my pocket, much to the chagrin of the charming lady standing in line behind me.

"Hello stranger," a familiar voice echoed in my ear.

"It's been awhile," I replied, returning my gaze to Ms. Cruz and those eyes.

"Thought you'd flown the coop," Carol said.

"I did. Right out of Faith General."

"We miss you."

"We?" I asked, easing my buggy forward to where I could unload.

"David and Jo have been asking about you."

"Tell them hello."

"That's it?" she asked.

"Yeah," I said as I greeted the check-out girl.

"Where are you?" Carol asked.

"You don't wanna know."

"Tell me anyway."

I was right. She didn't want to know that I had moved in with John and Maggie.

"Why?" Carol asked.

"They asked."

"You're kidding," Carol said. "What kind of deal...?"

"They're paying me and quite well," I said as I unloaded the remains of my grocery cart.

"To do what?" Carol asked. "You're not a nurse!"

"You're right, I'm not a nurse," I fired back as I slid the debit card through the machine. "I'm their friend," I said, hoping that my words hit home as I punched in my code number. "Beyond that, I'm part social worker, liaison, homemaker, caretaker and most importantly — confidante."

"I'm sorry," she replied, her tone mellowing. "I just don't understand."

"No, you don't," I abruptly agreed, angry that she had blown me off, as if what I was doing wasn't worthy. I saw it as the most precious and loving thing I'd done in a long, long time.

"Hey, I'm truly sorry," she said. "I just miss seeing you, okay?"

"You sure have a funny way of expressing it," I replied.

"Yeah, well…" She hesitated. "It's not like I've had that many opportunities to express my feelings here of late."

"Yes, they're paying me," I said, ignoring her dig, "but I don't care about the money and don't care if my life is put on hold for awhile. Six months seems minuscule in the grand scheme of things. If Maggie lasts that long."

"How's she doing?"

"Not good," I said, thanking the cashier. "She's hurting." I stashed the last bag in the buggy. "She never shows John the true extent of her gut-wrenching pain."

"Is she…?"

"Yeah, she's gonna die," I said as I teetered towards the car, "and probably sooner than expected."

"How long?"

"I don't know. She's not getting around like she was."

"How come her kids aren't there?"

"They didn't want to disrupt their lives," I said, opening the hatchback. "And honestly, there's a win-win-win in it for them."

"How so?" Carol asked.

"They get to stay in their home of fifty-plus years, their kids' lives are not turned upside down, and I needed a job."

"You're taking care of both of them by yourself?"

"Pretty much," I said, stuffing the groceries in the back. "I've got a home health nurse who comes in three times a week, and I'm building a network of volunteers and friends from their church. Even got a hospice nurse last week."

"Is she cute?"

"Who?"

"The home health nurse."

"Yes," I fired back, "but he's not my type."

"I'm sorry. I..."

"Can't understand why I'm doing this?" I said as I settled into my car. "Tell you what." I cranked the engine. "How 'bout next Tuesday at O'Charley's and I'll explain why."

"I'd like that very much."

"Me too," I replied as I exited the grocery store parking lot and headed for home. "Me too."

How do you explain to people that one day you're working as a crisis counselor in a psychiatric ER and the next day you're fired for helping an Alzheimer's patient escape, only to wind up taking care of him and his dying wife in exchange for room and board?

Maggie was deteriorating right before my eyes. The vibrant 74-year-old woman I'd met two months earlier was only a shell of that lovely lady, and yet somehow she mustered the courage every morning to stand with John in their rose garden. It was one of those rare moments that will remain etched in my mind, the two of them as one, talking and laughing, touching and caressing, a lifetime together amongst a bed of red, yellow, pink and white roses. And their favorite — a peach rose as divinely rich in color as their love and admiration for one another.

As I put the groceries up, I looked out across the lawn at two old people — Maggie knocking on death's door; John's mind slowly dead-bolting the door on reality as he perceived it. Neither afraid. Both with one final wish — to depart this world as one. Maggie in body, John in mind, their souls forever linked.

I wasn't sure how or even if such a wish could play out in their favor. And yet, as I waved to them from the kitchen window, I wasn't about to count them out. Not these two.

chapter thirty-four

"**Y**OU KNOW TO CALL ME," I said for the fifth time to John and Maggie.

"Go have a good time," John replied with a smile, "we'll be fine."

I backed out of their driveway, opened the moon roof, and located my favorite, classic rock radio channel, waiting, just as I had done as a seventeen-year-old, to crank the music up after departing the neighborhood, or in this case, the Dalton compound.

I sped towards the highway, feeling the breeze above, checking my phone to make sure it was on, hoping that my first real night away was, indeed, a joyous occasion.

It had been nearly nine weeks since I'd laid eyes on Carol. A lifetime in some ways, a fleeting moment in others. My life floated somewhere in the balance, as if caught in some time warp. Since moving in with John and Maggie, the outside world seemed a distant stranger. I spent my days cooking, cleaning, counseling, case managing, coaching, nursing, entertaining, financing and running errands. I monitored John's afternoon naps, making sure as best as I could that he woke up on the right side of reality. We hunkered down in the den most evenings after supper, John in his recliner, Maggie in her streamlined geri-chair right next to him, both content to watch baseball or Andy Griffith reruns.

I exited the interstate, the O'Charley's sign visible and a mere three minutes away. I coasted down to the red light, thinking what I wouldn't give for a second chance at love. I knew that Jenny was not the one. As intriguing and alluring as she remained in my mind, my heart knew better. We'd come together at a time when both of us were alone and connected to her parents.

Carol was a different story, a woman well aware of my cantankerous side, and yet who liked me in spite of such. "A rare woman indeed!" I mused as I pulled into the restaurant parking lot. I only hoped that the intimate friendship blossoming nine weeks ago hadn't wilted under an intense Dalton sky.

"You're looking good." Carol smiled.

"So do you," I lied. She looked beyond good. More like scrumptious in her tight-fitting jeans and wrap-top blue blouse cut teasingly low. Her brown hair hung freely down her back. Her face looked alive, sexy, artsy. Her smile and eyes spoke of an intense yet deeply caring soul. Here was the whole package, sitting directly across from me.

"You're blushing," she teased.

"Yeah, well I've been sequestered."

"Let me guess — an older woman," she hesitated, "or perhaps her daughter."

"No…" I went from blushing to frowning.

"Oops," she teased. "Sore spot huh?"

I ignored her comment as the waitress set our drinks down.

"So how are they doing?" Carol asked.

"Maggie's growing weaker." I glanced at the menu, then back at her. "And stronger too."

"In what way?"

"Her inner strength," I reached for the sugar packets, "and total commitment to John's well-being. I sweetened my tea. "She knows her pain will end soon and has no fear of death."

She leaned back, a teasing grin on her face as I stirred. "Still not sweet enough, huh?"

"Getting there," I smiled, feeling alive again, our sparring the fix I'd been craving.

"Is she in pain all the time?"

"Excruciating at times," I said. "She stays as clear-headed as possible during the morning hours." I picked the menu up. "They share their special time together."

She sipped her Margarita and looked at me, perplexed.

"What is it?" I asked.

She took another long swig and set her drink down. "It's just strange. Not bad, I don't mean this as bad strange."

"Some bad strange sounds good to me," I surmised.

"You've been locked up too long."

"No." I glanced around the restaurant, admiring the upbeat crowd. "The real problem is I'm addicted to derelicts and deranged souls, and… " I playfully held her gaze. "You're the first one I've talked to in three months."

"What?" she cried. "You want me to strip my clothes off and dance on the table?"

I grinned. "Now that definitely gets me the fix I need."

"You're sick old man," she fired back, her devilish smile and sexy charm never more appealing.

"I won't argue that point," I said. "So you were saying?"

Carol studied my face before continuing. "Michael, I've always admired your ability to interact comfortably with a variety of patients and staff and make them feel cared for."

"But… ?"

"You seemed so cold underneath all that charm," she said. "So distant and removed. Nobody could penetrate that wall. And then this old couple waltzes in one day…"

"And?"

She ran her finger lightly around the rim of her salted glass. "You go from being aloof and cantankerous to a man filled with compassion and love for his fellow man."

"What?" I squirmed in my seat. "You like me better as an asshole?"

She leaned back slowly, a sassy smile forming on her face. "I'm not sure."

I reached for my tea glass. "Sure makes me feel better." I took a long drink.

She leaned forward and placed her hand on my forearm. "I don't want to see you hurt. I worry about where you'll go and what you'll do. I miss working with you... " She looked up, her eyes misty. "I miss you."

"That's the best news I've heard in nine weeks," I said, touching her hand. "I was beginning to wonder if anybody missed me, or even cared for that matter."

"Poor David is lost without you."

"Yeah, you're probably making him see all of the borderlines."

"Of course," she said with a laugh.

"How's Jo doing?"

"She told me to tell you hello."

"She's good people."

We leaned back while the waiter set our desserts down and poured coffee. I looked up at Carol and smiled, happy to be with her, ecstatic that she still cared.

"Have you thought about life after Maggie and John?"

"Yes and no," I said as an unfamiliar vibration startled me.

"You okay?"

"My cell phone." I found my reading glasses and peered at the number on the screen. "I need to answer this," I apologized.

Carol graciously nodded.

A minute later I stashed the cell phone back in my pocket and stood. "I'm so sorry, but I have to go."

"Are you okay?" She reached for my hand. "Who is it?"

"Maggie. John won't go to bed and he's agitated."

"Shouldn't you call the police?"

"Maggie will hang in there." I reached for her hand.

"Is there anything I can do to help?"

"Yeah, don't give up on me."

chapter thirty-five

I PUSHED MY OLD HONDA TO its limit as I sped down the road, Carol's image fresh in my mind, along with racing thoughts about what I might be walking into in the next ten minutes.

I exited the highway and through the red light leading to their two-lane road. I glanced again at my phone, thinking that I'd heard it ring or beep. I tucked the cell phone between my legs and glued my eyes to the road, cutting off corners whenever possible in the black of night. I shook my head in disgust, angry that my date with Carol was cut short. "I'll call her," I murmured as I pulled into the Dalton driveway.

I jumped out of my car and scurried to the front door, unable to curb my racing thoughts. Why had I been so stupid to go out and leave them alone? Had John wandered off? Harmed Maggie? Why were all the lights off? I know I left the front porch light on, didn't I?

I eased my key into the lock, opened the front door, and tiptoed down the hall, an eerie silence engulfing me. I edged closer towards their bedroom, my forehead pulsating, my chest thumping. "Maggie?"

No answer.

I clutched the doorknob of their half-opened door and peeked in. "Maggie?" I called again, louder this time.

No sign of her.

"John!" I yelled as I quickly checked the other bedroom.

No sign or sound of either one of them!

"Oh man," I moaned, turning the empty bathroom light off. "Michael...?"

I heard a faint voice, perhaps from the kitchen. I ran down the hall.

"Michael?" Maggie called out. "Is that you?" Her sweet raspy voice soothed my raging heart.

"Out here on the porch!" called John, his voice sounding normal, even happy.

I flipped the porch light on. "You folks okay?" I asked as I flipped the lights back off and joined them.

"Like old times," John said. "Right, dear?"

"Quite a sight," she said, wrapped in a blanket on a muggy summer night, a tired smile on her hollow face.

I leaned forward, glancing at her. "You okay?"

"Fine," she nodded, winking at me as she held John's hand. "We woke up and couldn't go back to sleep. We're okay now," she said, her eyes telling me that she was sorry for ending my night so abruptly.

"That's good." I leaned back in my chair and took a long deep breath, relieved for their sake, saddened for mine.

chapter thirty-six

A s the summer heated up, the Dalton duo digressed along two dichotomous paths. Maggie's body was withering away, a mere skeleton of the woman I'd first met back in the spring. John's mind was fading away, the memory loss and increased confusion, especially at night, causing him to struggle with seemingly simple tasks. Neither was able to manage alone, and yet, together, they somehow functioned as one, Maggie lending her mind to her man, John using his body to help move her about.

Jenny and Matthew made frequent visits over the summer. I usually stayed in the background after giving basic instructions on managing the household and the steady flow of medical staff, volunteers and friends on any given day. It was amazing to watch Maggie and John put on a show for their children, fighting every step of the way to make things appear upbeat and okay. For the most part they pulled it off.

As they departed each time, both Matthew and Jenny commented on how well Mom and Dad were doing. As soon as one or the other left, Mom and Dad fell apart. Until the next weekend visit. Before long, it became a standing bet between Maggie and me as to whether or not Matthew or Jenny would recognize the extent of their decline. Most of the time they either didn't or played their own game of hide-and-seek with the truth. Whatever the case, both Jenny and Matthew routinely called me once they made it back home to get my scoop. I played both sides of the fence, not an easy task for even the slickest of mental health veterans.

As the summer came to a close and the lush green trees prepared for their annual fall curtain call, there was little left for Maggie to hide. She seldom ventured far from her bedside perch in the den, her frail body no longer able to sit up for extended periods of time. Much of her time was spent in and out of sleep due to the increased need for medications to soothe the excruciating pain. And yet, she still managed to spend quality time with John during the mid-morning hours when he was more lucid and lighthearted.

They called it their special time. The two lovebirds would gaze at pictures and relive old memories, a history lesson of their lives together. It didn't matter to Maggie that she retold the same stories every morning. It didn't matter to him that she sometimes dozed off in the middle of one of her tales. He'd sit and gently stroke her face and forehead until she came to again, picking back up with her story and never missing a beat. Of course, John had already forgotten the part she'd told him not five minutes earlier, and Maggie would revel in the chance to walk down memory lane again with the man she so dearly loved.

It evolved into a beloved time for me as well. Before John awoke, I'd spruce Maggie up as best as I could, dabbing a bit of make-up here and there to make her feel special. Afterwards, she'd always ask me to read from Psalms or one of her daily devotionals. We'd cover every meaningful subject under the sun. In our world, the only meaningful subjects were the three of us and our kids, and grandkids in Maggie's case. Nothing else mattered to her, and frankly, to me either.

Despite her decaying body and sometimes fog-filled mind, her spirit and inner fire were very much alive. Maggie, the dying cancer patient, became Maggie, my therapist, teacher, and mother figure. She challenged me to find "my calling" as she liked to say, after my time with them was over. She emphatically told me that I'd been called to do what I was doing now, and the two of them would be eternally grateful for the sacrifices I'd made. However, my spiritual journey was only beginning, not ending with their deaths. It was indeed a very special time, those precious minutes with her. Beyond her surrogate roles as counselor, mentor and mother figure, she was, above all, my friend.

John and I had our moments together too. As Maggie dozed, he and I played simple card games and continued our on-going feud regarding Mays, the Mick (Mantle), and DiMaggio. Nary a day went by that he didn't ask about my son and what I was doing to rectify the situation. Those were the good days, sharing walks and talks and ballgames on the boob tube.

Then there were the days when things weren't so good. He loved to sit at the kitchen table while I cooked. One minute he'd be fine, talking to me in the present and understanding my responses. The next minute, however, he'd repeat himself over and over, oblivious to our conversation only minutes earlier.

His delusional episodes remained manageable as long as I gently woke him up from his naps and assured him of his surroundings. He did remarkably well when we'd take trips to the store or run household errands. I'd take him with me while the hospice nurse sat with Maggie. There was the one time we got separated in the grocery store and John wound up with a buggy-full of diapers and baby food to take home to his two toddlers. And then there was the ordeal in the bank a few weeks ago when he argued with the startled teller that she'd given him too much money.

As the fall colors filled the surrounding hills with lush reds and bright oranges, John's short-term memory virtually disappeared, as if conversations and events less than five minutes old never happened. Interesting enough, his long-term memory remained sharp. His demeanor grew surly when he couldn't understand what was happening around him or complete simple tasks like answering the phone or changing TV channels. Yet, he rarely displayed his anger in Maggie's presence and never forgot who she was.

In the late afternoon, I'd often sit with him on the back deck or monitor him from the kitchen window while I cooked supper. He scared me one time. I'd gone to the bathroom, only to find him missing from view upon my return. I bolted out the back door and towards the woods where I found him halfway up the tree house. Amidst a sea of orange, we enjoyed an Indian summer sunset in the tree house as John told me the story of building his penthouse in the sky with remarkable clarity. He told me five times.

As we strolled back to the house at dusk that day, he shared a heartfelt plan he'd devised, a remarkable plan, given his current condition, one that required my participation if it were to work.

The following morning started like any other as Maggie and I finished our special time together. John took his seat next to her while I retrieved several picture albums. I watched from the kitchen as they took their customary stroll down memory lane, Maggie patiently retelling the events of days gone by.

"Oh look," Maggie said, "that's us at the beach." She pointed to the picture, her eyes alive.

John looked down at the picture deadpanned.

I edged closer to them, wondering if this was the moment.

"John..." Maggie's bony right hand reached out to him. "You okay?"

John held her gaze momentarily, his face softening, his eyes filling with tears. "I love you."

"I love you too," she whispered, her raspy voice tiring.

"I'm so sorry," he cried, "I can't do this."

"Do what, honey?" She gently stroked his haggard face.

He laid his head down on her shoulder. No words were shared, the two as one, John unable to follow through with his heartfelt plan. A plan that troubled me, but I'd blest.

chapter thirty-seven

As the fall foliage fell to the cold damp ground, Maggie clung to life and the hope that John's memory of her would fade away. John was indeed fading, yet he was focused enough to feel Maggie's immense pain and suffering. That's why he'd wanted so desperately to follow-through with his plan but couldn't bear the thought of deceiving her. Honesty had worked for fifty-six years. Why stoop to deceit now? And yet, he didn't have the heart to tell her, nor was he ready to face life without her.

As it turned out, Maggie was feeling his pain too. I watched the story unfold, wanting desperately to intervene in some way. It was a mid-November morn, unseasonably warm, uncharacteristically early for Maggie to be calling for me. I was sitting in the kitchen reading and sipping coffee. John was still fast asleep.

"You okay?" I asked, her eyes troubled and tired.

"What was John referring to the other day?"

"When?" I patted her face down with a soft towel.

"When he told me he was sorry he couldn't do it."

I hesitated, not wanting to break confidence with him. He'd shared his innermost thoughts and desires, and I wasn't one to discuss the secrets of another. Maggie, however, sensed my uneasiness. Four months of living together and sharing our innermost feelings qualified her hunch.

She squeezed my hand. "I've got to know if what I'm thinking is right."

"You tell me," I replied with a smile.

She knew exactly what John was thinking. She just couldn't pinpoint his specific plan of action. Under the circumstances, I decided to tell her.

"And he thought I wouldn't know?" she asked, the troubled look fading away.

"He wasn't sure," I said, "but he can't stand seeing you in such pain."

"Why did he stop?" she asked.

"You tell me," I said, "you're batting a thousand so far." I laid my hand on her forehead. "Besides, I think you know him pretty well by now."

"Yes..." She pulled me in closer, her frail bony finger touching my cheek, her hazel eyes alive with delight. "Yes, indeed."

I sat beside her, my forearms dangling across the side rail of her hospital bed. We sat in silence, seemingly lost in the moment.

She closed her eyes and smiled. "Thank-you Michael."

"Not a word." I leaned over and kissed her on her cheek.

"Not a word," she whispered with a childlike smile.

John never knew that Maggie knew. His defunct plan had been simple, the love and courage behind it only fifty-six years of marriage could fathom. He had planned to fake a memory lapse, the most painful of lapses — pretending that he didn't recognize Maggie. A frightening notion for a man with a disease that had already stripped him of his short term memory and would one day wipe out every recollection he'd ever had of family, friend, or foe. He dreaded that day, and yet, in a strange way, longed for it, knowing his voided life would yield a pain-free bounty for Maggie.

Till death do us part...

John's mind.

Maggie's body.

If he no longer recognized her, there was nothing to stop her from letting go. And yet, as much as he longed for her pain and suffering to end, he couldn't bear lying to her. He had told me in tears later that afternoon. "I just couldn't look her in the eye and lie."

I decided to intervene on their behalf. Truth be known, the idea came from a higher authority. I'd spent the past three late nights in the tree house trying to figure out what I could do, to no avail. How else do you explain rising up in bed at four in the morning with a crystal- clear picture of what needed to happen?

chapter thirty-eight

I WATCHED FROM THE DALTON KITCHEN as daylight slowly emerged from the darkness. The giant oak tree cradling the tree house out back stood leafless and naked amidst a cold gray sky. I flipped Maggie's TV on and turned it to the Weather Channel. The forecast for the weekend called for more of the same, with the threat of sleet, possibly even snow. I turned the TV off and sipped my coffee, savoring the silence of the moment, the only sound in the house the ticking of an old grandfather clock that stood alone in the seldom used living room. I grabbed my planning folder and rechecked every item on the list, still worried that I might have left something out.

I walked out onto the deck and called Jenny, hoping that she'd be up, Asheville on Eastern Time.

"What happens if the weather is bad?" she asked.

"It's a go, come rain or shine," I said, surveying the bleak sky first hand from the dampened back deck. "What time's your flight?"

"We're driving over in the morning. I'm bringing the kids for this."

"Wonderful!" I said. "Matthew's kids are coming too." I

glanced at my watch. "I'm picking them up at the airport later this afternoon."

"Mom will be so pleased that all of her grandkids will be there."

"Your father is excited too," I said, wanting to tell her that John's exuberance repeated itself every few minutes, but I opted otherwise.

"Pray for sunshine," she said. "See you tomorrow."

"I can't wait."

By ten in the morning, my to-do list was coming to life, including an extra set of volunteer hands due to arrive any minute. I had to go to the grocery store and pick out our roast and all of the fixings, not to mention the ingredients I would need to make John's favorite dessert — pineapple upside down cake, my first attempt at such. I was on my own in the kitchen, although my cooking coach and confidante would be available for questions if I ran into problems.

I whizzed around the grocery store, checking off items as I found them. I glanced at my watch again, ever mindful of making sure the flower arrangement, with its centerpiece of peach roses, was ready to be delivered as planned.

I sped through the check-out line, oblivious this trip to the end-of-time predictions splattered across the headlines of my favorite tabloid. I hustled out to the car, loaded the groceries, and climbed into the driver's seat, the late-fall blast of bone-chilling air reeking havoc with my aching back.

As I prepared to back out, my phone rang. It was Matthew, touching base from Dallas where he and his family were changing planes. "We're right on schedule," he told me.

"Wish I could say the same," I muttered as I hung up. I slid the car into reverse, only to put it back in park as I glanced down at my phone. I looked around the parking lot, relieved that what few shoppers were out this morning appeared unaware of me. I held my phone up to where I could see it without my reading glasses. I dialed my son's number but hung up before it rang, painfully aware that the more I forced my way into his life, the more he resisted returning my calls. I glanced around the parking lot, wondering if Carol was up and painting this morning. I leaned back in my seat, recalling our night out awhile back and how good she looked, my insides tingling at the thought of her touch.

I dialed the first four digits of her number, only to hang up. I tossed the phone on the passenger seat and pulled out of the parking lot, hoping that when the time came, Carol would give me one more shot. "Just not tomorrow."

⤛⤜

I stood in the Dalton kitchen at two in the morning, the only sound the mesmerizing ticking of the grandfather clock. I felt like I was ten years old again on the eve of my first Little League baseball game. I couldn't sleep for fear of oversleeping, the anticipation and excitement running rampant in my mind. I quietly reached into the refrigerator freezer, the thought of low-fat, heavenly hash, frozen yogurt soothing to my stomach. I devoured the remains of the half-gallon tub as I gazed out the window.

I grabbed an old jacket from the utility closet and ventured out onto the deck. I stood in the cold mist, nary a star or the moon in sight, the blackened sky thick with fog and clouds. My thoughts flashed back to the day we buried my father. I shivered and then laughed as I recalled that bitter cold snowy afternoon sixteen years ago. As we rode out to the burial site in a Hearst, my Mom, brothers and I all snickered and agreed that Pop got his wish. He wasn't one to want a bunch of people making a fuss over him.

I shivered one last time and glanced skyward. *Put in a word for blue sky, Pop.*

—⟶🙰

I flitted about the kitchen, thrilled that my roast was moist and tasty, amazed that the pineapple upside down cake survived my attempt. Actually, I cheated, giving way to Betty Crocker's recipe, the fear factor of screwing it up from scratch too strong. I did throw in fresh cut pineapple.

"Hey!" I called out as Jenny burst into the kitchen looking sexy and stylish in her form fitting sweater and jeans.

She gave me a warm hug and introduced me to her college-aged girls, who were fast to exit the kitchen in search of their California cousins.

"Can you believe this?" Jenny said. "Nothing but sleet and fog coming across the mountains and all the way through Knoxville." She opened the oven door and peeked in. "Um, that smells good. Any chance I can hire you out?"

I smiled back at her, the first relaxed moment I could recall of this day. "I'm going to need some time off when this gig is up," I said. "Although..." I hesitated and took a long deep breath as Matthew wandered in. "It's been an experience I'll savor for the rest of my life."

"Am I interrupting?" Matthew asked.

"Oh no," I said, "Jenny was telling me about her trip over the mountains."

"You made it, huh?" Matthew said as he gave her a bear hug.

"We crossed the Cumberland Plateau and the sky opened up, the temperature rose, and now this — a Carolina blue sky and temperatures near sixty. Is everyone here?" she asked.

"The entire crew," Matthew said.

"Mom and Dad?" she asked, sounding timid. "They okay?"

"Excited," I said, "nervous, but ready. How 'bout you guys?"

"We're ready," Jenny replied as she draped her arm around Matthew and led him outside to where their kids and Matthew's wife had gathered on the deck.

"Me too," I said, glancing skyward. "Thanks Pop."

chapter thirty-nine

AN OLD COUNTRY CHURCH STOOD alone in a field, surrounded by rolling hills. A small graveyard was tucked away out back, a giant oak tree on either end standing guard. A lily-white steeple high atop a bell tower stretched skyward. The smell of pine and cedar permeated the tiny sanctuary. The old pulpit from which fire and brimstone had once spewed down upon the congregation had long-since succumbed to silence. You didn't need a preacher to feel the spirit of the Almighty on this day.

Fifty-six years ago, they stood as one in this same sanctuary. Fifty-six years later, John and Maggie Dalton were hand-in-hand again, Maggie exerting every ounce of energy left in her listless body to sit upright in a wheelchair. John sat by her side, ever so proud, ever so humble, fighting to hang on to reality just one more time.

They were surrounded by family — a son and daughter-in-law, a daughter, and five granddaughters, all old enough to grasp that what they were about to witness would stay with them for a lifetime.

One minister.

A choir of three.

A small gathering of friends.

One privileged guest – me, sitting in the back, a myriad of emotions stirring within.

All gathered to celebrate the lives of John and Maggie Dalton, a few honored to share their favorite memories and stories destined to grow in stature over time among the Dalton gang. As the laughter faded from the final tale spun by their longtime next-door neighbor and dear friend, the minister approached the pulpit.

"John Robert Dalton, do you take this woman to be your wedded wife for eternity? To have and to hold from this day forward until the day you reunite in heaven?"

"I do."

"Margaret Louise Dalton, do you take this man to be your wedded husband for eternity? To have and to hold from this day forward until the day you reunite in heaven?"

"I do."

"Who giveth this woman permission to pass on from this lifetime to God's infinite love and heavenly home?"

"We do..." John stood and gingerly turned his bride towards their offspring, who collectively nodded and smiled through their tears.

The grandkids approached one at a time and said good-bye. Maggie presented each with a keepsake. Jenny approached, then Matthew, both sharing a private moment with their mother as John slumped teary-eyed by her side, overcome with emotion.

"Let us pray."

The four of them, John and Maggie, Jenny and Matthew, hunkered down on the front pew, entwined as one in embrace.

"Heavenly Father, we beseech you to free Maggie from her earthly pain and suffering so that she may join you. Father, we also ask that you bless John. Give him the strength to live out his days with the sweet knowledge that one day he and Maggie will be joined again as one."

A voice softly rang out, soon joined by two. Three heavenly voices, as sweet and clear as I've ever heard, sang their heartfelt rendition of Amazing Grace as the Dalton kids and grandkids gathered around John and Maggie one last time.

I felt a tingling in my heart, the warmest of feelings as I wept in the back of that old country church. God wasn't just looking down on us today. He was here.

Ready to take one of his children home.

chapter forty

IT HAD BEEN TWO WEEKS since the church ceremony and things at the Dalton compound were back to normal. Matthew and Jenny had returned home with their families. Both wanted to stay, perhaps expecting the inevitable sooner than later, however John and Maggie would have no part of it, making it painfully clear that they were paying me to take care of them and did not want their kids saddled with any of the responsibilities, no matter how much Matthew and Jenny insisted.

Maggie also had a hospice nurse monitoring her condition throughout the day while John and I sat with her during the evening hours. I had taken to sitting up with her throughout much of the night as well, at times doing nothing more than cradling her hand while she dozed, her breathing becoming shallower with each passing day.

It was late Wednesday afternoon, two weeks before Thanksgiving. Maggie had mustered the energy to speak to both of her kids via phone, letting them know that all was well. Of course, each asked to speak to me immediately afterwards. I played the good employee, as instructed by my boss, and shared only minimal information with Matthew and Jenny. However, I encouraged them to read between the lines and book a flight.

On the following day, John's weekly flower arrangement arrived right on time. Following the church ceremony, John had approached me about ordering his bride flowers every Thursday. John couldn't wait to show them to Maggie. He gently shooed the hospice nurse away for a few minutes. I watched from the kitchen, the glow on Maggie's face at the sight of her beaming beau with his bouquet of peach roses as pure a picture of love as I have ever seen; the two of them living in the moment and fearless in the face of death.

It was later that same night, actually a few minutes after midnight, as I snoozed in my chair next to Maggie, that I felt a squeeze of my hand.

"Can you raise my bed a bit?" she whispered.

I sat up, shaking my head to clear the cobwebs. "You bet." I grabbed the magic buttons. "Tell me when."

She smiled, reaching up to adjust the oxygen cannula leading into each nostril. "That's good. Thank you." She laid her head back and took a deep breath.

"How you feeling?" I asked, leaning forward to touch her shoulder.

"About as good as I look," she said. "Is John okay?"

"Sleepin' like a baby," I said, "and snoring like a freight train."

Maggie reached up and patted my hand, her smile and those emerald eyes still captivating. "How are you holding up?"

I smiled at her. "I'm okay."

She studied my face, her cold frail hand grasping mine. "Have you heard from your son?"

I looked away momentarily. "Not yet."

She caressed my hand the way a mother soothes her child. "He'll come around." She took a breath, her eyes exuding genuine warmth and compassion. "Don't you give up hope."

I nodded and smiled. "I won't."

We sat in silence for a moment, lost in thought amid the quiet that surrounded us.

"Can I get you anything?" I asked.

She took a breath, and then smiled. "Read to me."

"Psalms?"

"The Apostle Paul," she said.

"Any preference?"

"Your pick."

I flipped to First Corinthians, chapter 13, cleared my throat and read. "If I speak in the tongues of men and of angels, but have not love, I am only a resounding gong or clanging cymbal."

Maggie closed her eyes, a smile shaping her sunken face.

I read. "If I have the gift of prophecy and can fathom all mysteries... If I give all I possess to the poor and surrender my body to the flames, but have not love, I gain nothing."

I continued, Maggie reciting parts of verses with me. "Love is patient, love is kind. It does not envy, it does not boast... Love never fails..."

As I came to the final verse of chapter 13, radiance filled the room, emitting warmth that penetrated deep within me. "And now these three remain," I read, "faith, hope and love." I glanced at Maggie before reading the last line, her eyes reflecting a deep peace. "But the greatest of these is love."

I set the Bible down and reached for her hand. Her breathing slowed, her face softened, and her eyes sparkled as we bask in the silence of the night and the glow of the room.

chapter forty-one

I PULLED UP TO THE SPANKING new facility on the outskirts of town, just as I had done every Sunday and during the weeks over the past month. I eased out of my car and hustled inside to the locked doors leading in. I punched in the four digit code and walked down the hallway leading to John's new home.

"You got this place looking good," I said as I shook John's hand. "And of course, your beloved Lazy Boy."

"It's okay," he replied, "I won't be here long."

"Why's that?" I asked.

"Just a feeling," he said, void of any emotion.

"A feeling?" I sat across from him.

"What day is this?" he asked.

"Sunday, December 18th. Why?"

"Is this the day you said you'd be here?"

"Of course," I said, "I told you on Wednesday that I'd be back today, just like I have every Sunday..." I stopped, not wanting to upset him anymore than he already appeared. "So what's this feeling?"

"What feeling?" John snapped.

"You said that you had a feeling you wouldn't be here long."

"I wasn't referring to this place," he replied, a twinkle in his eye.

"Are you going to tell me, or do I have to pull it out of you?" I teased.

Alzheimer's is indeed a strange disease. Since Maggie's death four weeks ago, his condition had worsened. He'd immediately moved out of the house and into an assisted living complex for Alzheimer's, the abruptness catching me off guard. I soon found out that he and Maggie had worked out a back-up plan, which, as previously agreed upon, still included me as the power of attorney for healthcare for John.

In retrospect, it made perfect sense. I remember John telling me the day after Maggie died at home that he had to get out of there, that he didn't belong in their house without Maggie by his side. As expected, his symptoms worsened; the memory loss, confusion, and inability to perform routine daily tasks faded away and fast. On top of that, he was severely depressed, still mourning Maggie's death. The surprising and strange part of his illness — amidst the deterioration and devastation, he would still have moments when his mind was right on, his memory of our time together vivid and clear.

John leaned back in his old chair, the only furniture holdover from home. Home was now a one-bedroom apartment minus the kitchen. It was small but clean, adequate arrangements for a man teetering in and out of an Alzheimer's fog.

"After Maggie died..." He hesitated, struggling to keep his composure. "I kept asking God to take me."

"And?" I leaned forward.

"Obviously," he said with a smile, "He had something left for me to do."

"Any ideas?" I asked.

"For the longest time, no," he said. "My kids are fine,

grandkids too. I don't have any other family. I had no idea what God wanted me to do."

I nodded, holding eye contact with him.

He said, "I got my answer a couple of weeks ago."

"In the form of?" I asked, curious as to where he was going with his story.

"What?" He looked at me perplexed, and for a brief moment I was afraid I'd lost him.

"How'd God tell you?" I asked.

"He just told me!" he snapped.

"Told you what?" I asked, intrigued.

John slowly sat up, a fatherly look on his face. "Well," he said, "it took some work, and both Jenny and Matthew helped me out." He struggled to stand but made it on his own.

I stood next to him. "The suspense is…" I stopped as a loud knock wrapped on his door. "You expecting someone?" I asked.

John grinned. "Right on time. Go ahead, open it."

I obliged.

"Hello Pop," said a voice that I hadn't heard in a long time.

"Kind of favors a young Joe DiMaggio, don't you think?" John said. "Sure is better lookin' than his old man."

I grabbed my son in the doorway and hugged him. "Can't argue with that."

epilogue

THREE MONTHS LATER, THE ER nurse snapped. "You expecting James Patterson?"

"Never heard of him," I replied, glancing at our referral board. "What's the scoop?"

"Eighty-one-year-old shooting up mailboxes," she said blasé. "Thinks his wife's hiding men in there."

"Is she with him?" I asked, reaching for an assessment packet.

"Sweet as she can be."

"I'll be out in a minute."

It feels good to be back home. There's something about this ER that grows on me, a bad analogy since the March weather has turned bipolar-like, lending itself to a variety of flu and icky viruses. Whatever the case, I'm back! Faith General's ivory tower turned over, and Dr. Qualls grew weary of being Baxter's pawn, prompting Baxter's move back east.

I was fortunate that Jo was still running our office. I don't know what cock-and-bull story she told the new CEO. Something about I was off my meds the day I transported John across hospital lines to freedom. Whatever the case, I signed a pre-employment agreement that if the urge hit me to kidnap another patient, I'd immediately call a code one hundred and allow hospital staff to restrain me.

David was thrilled that I'd come back to lend a hand. The female, borderline, bipolar contingent had swelled in numbers over the winter. Something about being cooped up with their football-crazed men.

Carol? She's still around. An intimate friend and psych ER comrade. A gifted painter. And the morning light in her studio? My old visions don't hold a candle to a box seat view of her dabbling in briefs.

My son and I made up for lost time, thanks to John. Apparently he and Matthew worked my boy over pretty good. John told him that I'd sacrificed my job and life for him and Maggie and any man willing to do that deserved a second chance. Apparently John's version of the great escape and subsequent reunion with Matthew was the kicker that coerced my son to drive to Nashville. It was the greatest Christmas gift I've ever received — my son's forgiveness. We converse weekly now. Even spent a few weekends together. Turns out he likes to dance and loves coming to Nashville to kick up his boot heels. Oh, the days when I could do some serious two-steppin...

I think about John and Maggie quite often and how they entered my life at a time when I was desperate for a purpose, a focus, an awakening. Last Christmas was John's last. He died peacefully one cold January morn a mere two months after Maggie departed this earth. John was one of the lucky ones, you might say — passing in his sleep, escaping the slow, decaying death sentence of Alzheimer's.

The last time I saw him was New Year's Eve. We took a ride together for old time's sake. Cruised the Faith General parking lot laughing all the way. Even drove by his old house and Maggie's grave. He told her he was ready now and sure hoped it wouldn't be long because he missed her.

When we got back to his apartment, he shooed me away. Said I needed to be with Carol on the last day of the year. I argued with him. Told him Carol didn't get off work till ten. It didn't matter. He ran me out anyway, but not before one final surprise. We had one last argument about Mays and Mantle. Then he brought up the Yankee Clipper, Joe DiMaggio. Said he was the greatest, and I was the only person left who could truly appreciate how good Joltin' Joe was.

I got that old autographed baseball of John's sitting right next to my computer screen at home. When I sit down to surf the internet or e-mail my son, my eye always catches that baseball. Joe DiMaggio's fifty-six game hitting streak is still in the record books seventy-plus years later. Some say the Yankee Clipper's record will never be broken. I can't help but think about John and Maggie's record when I hold that ball in my hands.

I'm not sure when the good guys go to heaven, but I do believe one thing with all my heart — I can't imagine a heaven without the likes of John and Maggie Dalton.

One day I hope to find out.

And if Mays, the Mick and DiMaggio are all up there, maybe we'll settle our argument for good.

acknowledgments

Going back to 1998, when I wrote this novel, there have been many family members, friends, and coworkers who have read and provided valuable feedback. I am grateful to them all. A special thanks goes to my brother, Tom, who has read every rewrite of this story since 1998, and to Alexander von Ness at www.nessgraphica.com for the cover design.

Donna, my wife, has been there throughout, both as supporter of my writing and as a coworker. When I first started working in a psychiatric emergency room in 1996, even though I had 20 years mental health experience, I had never worked directly with the elderly and was frightened by them, given that many had comorbid medical complications. An exceptional nurse with experience across multiple medical and psychiatric settings, Donna took me under her angelic wing. As my fear of evaluating the elderly faded, my fondness for them grew, their stories often deeply touching me. I'm honored to have had the privilege of interviewing them.

I started my writing journey in the mid-1990s. By 2009, I had five unpublished novels on the shelf and the first draft of a memoir about my mental health journey. I came to my senses, sought professional help, and met Lisa Dale Norton on a whim at the annual Southern Festival of Books in Nashville. An acclaimed memoirist, former writing instructor at UCLA, and seasoned editor, she agreed to work with me. The best analogy I can offer, given that I live in the Music City is: I was a self-taught fiddle player, who was given the incredible opportunity to work with a classically educated and trained violinist. Lisa and I were eight months into my memoir when John and Maggie Dalton started calling my name 12 years after I had created them. Lisa agreed to work with me on the rewrite of this novel. I'm blest to work with her and look forward to returning to that memoir soon.

BIRDCAGE
www.midnightbirdcage.com

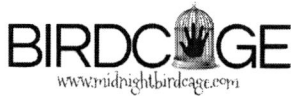

tales from a psychiatric ER...

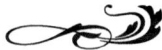

Wisdom is often times nearer when we stoop than when we soar.

Wordsworth

I STAND OUTSIDE OF THE SIDE entrance with my employee badge in hand, primed to key the wall lock that opens the steel-enforced security door leading into the psychiatric ER and my upcoming 12-hour shift. I take a deep breath, mutter my mantra ("Showtime..."), and grasp the door handle, hoping that our locked-down dungeon of a day hall is empty, yet anticipating that there will be eyes watching me as I enter. Some sad and suicidal, a level of hopelessness seemingly beyond repair; others manic and labile, oblivious to the madness racing through their chemically imbalanced brains; still others demented or demon possessed, or perhaps just good ol' boy inebriated eyes craving a smoke and another shot of liquid sustenance.

I scurry past an empty day room and unlock the door leading into the Birdcage, AKA our psych assessments office. The front and side walls of the Birdcage are primarily Plexiglas, providing staff the much-needed capability to monitor our patients' every move in the hallway. Unfortunately, the Plexiglas allows patients the opportunity to watch us as well, oft-times glaring, their noses nearly touching our see-through office walls in their never-ending attempts to rush us along.

"So what did I do to deserve this?" I ask my co-workers, thrilled that the day room is empty and no patients are waiting to be assessed.

"You wish…" they reply in unison, pointing to our referral board where I see a female name on the board as having just arrived out front.

"How wild?" I ask.

I don't have to wait for an answer. I hear a commotion rolling down the outside hallway and cuss under my breath, the rumbling female voice, like rapids on a river, growing louder, slowly building to a roar, stirring butterflies deep within my belly.

"Susie's in the house," Barry muses, turning towards me. "Your favorite kind of patient," he says, handing me the referral paperwork.

"Big and bad to the bone," Donna says, smiling.

I glare at my teammates. "Payback is mine."

I scan the crisis team's faxed description of her behavior — labile, agitated, pacing, openly arguing with herself, at one point telling crisis staff that God had told her she was the chosen one to lead the revolution and, "ain't a damn thing anybody gonna do to stop me…" In addition, group home staff where Susie resides reported that she stopped taking her meds a week ago and had grown increasingly agitated over the past few days, culminating in the assault of another resident, prompting their police call earlier in the day.

When schizophrenics stop taking their meds and become psychotic and agitated, one way to safely subdue them is a chemical cocktail such as Haldol and Ativan together in a one-shot syringe. When that same schizophrenic is two-hundred-and-fifty-plus pounds and stout, as in Susie's case, with a history of unprovoked assaults on staff and peers, the risk factor skyrockets in a free-standing psych ER where there is no on-site medical ER and immediate access to a physician. Translation — We got no meds. Just our wits...

I step out into our hallway where Susie paces. I approach her slowly. "What's happening Susie," I say, lo-key.

She turns and sizes me up, her chest expanding. She crosses her arms and glares at me, her eyes as dark as her chocolate-colored skin, her oversized blue sweatshirt thick, yet not dense enough to hide the hideous fact that her massive breasts are unrestrained by a bra.

I ease in closer to her, hoping to make a connection, and not of the left hook variety. "My name's Joe." I look down for a moment then back up, all cylinders firing in my spindly legs, ready to move if she lunges at me. "I'm one of the assessment..."

"I know who you are," she growls.

"You hungry?" I ask, ignoring her comment.

"What you got?" She starts towards me.

I nonchalantly turn to walk with her, again ignoring her passive threat to see if I'll flinch. "We usually got ham or turkey sandwiches and chips," I say. "Might even find a coke or sprite."

She walks on by me on her way to the other end of the hallway. "You got mayonnaise?" she asks, never bothering to turn around.

"I'll find you some," I say.

"Git me ham..."

"Comin' right up," I say.

I open the Birdcage door, slide over to the back portion where the miniscule patient refrigerator sits, and grab a ham sandwich sack, complete with chips and a cup of fruit. I fill a Styrofoam cup with Coke, nudge the frig door closed with my knee and start back out the door.

Donna flags me down.

I let her know who's at the top of my food chain at the moment and hustle back out into the hallway. "Where you wanna eat?" I ask Susie.

She stops pacing and looks at me from the other end of the hallway.

I ease towards her, sandwich bag and drink in hand. "You wanna watch TV while you eat, or sit over here in the big blue chair?"

She starts mumbling to herself, cursing.

I set her food down on one of the chairs facing the TV. "Make yourself at home." I step away from her food. "If you need anything, let me know," I say. "I'm working on getting you upstairs."

Susie plops down and tears into the food bag. She struggles to get her sandwich open, an excessive amount of plastic wrapped around it.

"Here…" I ease down on one knee, take the sandwich from her and unwrap it. "Okay?" I nod, opening her potato chip bag.

She glances at me, then grabs her sandwich and devours an entire half in two bites.

I stand up, gently pat her shoulder, and let her know that I'll check on her shortly. I start towards the office.

"Mista Joe," Susie calls out.

I spin back around. "Yes ma'am."

"Can I git another sandwich?"

"You sure can," I say and head for the frig.

"What I wanted to tell you," Donna says as I start back out again.

"Yeah…" I gesture as I unwrap another sandwich, hand it to Susie, and slide back onto my Birdcage perch.

"Dr. Ayottolah called."

"He's not on call," I say. "Is he still here?"

"He was," she says.

"Was?" I turn towards her.

"He called right before you came in," she says. "I'd asked him to stop by on his way out to sign the second committal on Susie so we could get her moved upstairs."

"And…?"

"That was him on the phone, saying that he forgot to stop by."

"Is he coming back?" I ask as I sign onto the computer.

"He's already halfway home."

"He's what?" I say, reaching for the phone.

"Who are you calling?"

"The units." I look up and see Susie content for the moment.

"I've already called," Donna says.

"Any other docs still around?" I ask, already sensing the answer from the look on her face.

"Not a one."

"Son of a…" I mumble under my breath as I glance at my watch.

"That's not even the bad news," Donna says, then turns to Barry, sitting at his usual post to our right.

"The ER just called," he says. "They won't make an exception to the 7p rule."

"What?" I cry. "You're kidding?"

"I wish…"

I shake my head in disgust as I complete Susie's assessment in the computer. Our pressing problem — We have a patient who needs to be committed involuntarily, all of our psychiatrists are gone for the day, and our back-up plan, our parent (medical) hospital's ER, has a no-committal time zone from 3p.m. to 7p.m. whereby we can't transfer involuntary patients for the ER MD's to evaluate and commit to our facility for an evaluation. The ER docs argue that our psychiatrists should be responsible during that time period. Sounds good on paper, until a situation like today arises when, like most days, our psychiatrists have all departed by three, and a psychotic and potentially violent patient arrives in need of a second involuntary committal paper, which can only be signed by a MD. It's one thing for us to hold a patient for an hour or so until such time the patient can be sent to the ER. Even then, an hour without any way of medicating a potentially violent psychotic patient is risky business. To maintain that same type of patient in our setting for four hours?

"So what do we do?" Donna asks.

I hit the print button and stand. "It'll take somebody getting maimed down here…" I turn and walk back out into the hallway. "You get enough to eat?" I ask Susie.

She looks up at me and appears to nod, although I'm not positive.

"I'll be right back, okay? I got some papers for you to sign, and then I can walk you upstairs where you get your own room. That sound okay?"

She looks at me again, this time nodding ever so slightly.

I return to the Birdcage and call the admissions clerk, letting her know that Susie is ready to be admitted. She thinks I'm crazy when I say voluntary (vs. involuntary) admission. I hang the phone up and see Barry and Donna gawking at me.

"You got any better ideas?" I snap.

They look at each other and then back at me.

I start towards the office door. "You want to do the honors?" I ask Barry.

"Oh no…" He laughs. "She likes you."

"Donna?" I gesture.

"I wouldn't do that to her," she says, playfully batting her eyelashes.

"Yeah, right…" I start out the door.

"Have fun," my comrades tease.

I ignore them as I turn my focus to the task at hand —

convincing Susie to sign the admission papers. Otherwise, we'll be stuck monitoring her for the next four hours without meds to give her, cigarettes to subdue her, or Jerry Springer on the boob tube to divert her.

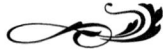

For the conclusion to this chapter one story, "Sign on the Boob Line…" and other stories from the Birdcage, go to midnightbirdcage.com, or joemichaelpritchard.com.

CPSIA information can be obtained
at www.ICGtesting.com
Printed in the USA
LVOW12s2252191116
513777LV00001B/41/P